Water Yoga

WATER YOGA

A Teacher's Guide to Improving
Movement, Health, and Wellbeing

CHRISTA FAIRBROTHER

Foreword by Ruth Sova

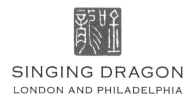

SINGING DRAGON
LONDON AND PHILADELPHIA

First published in Great Britain in 2022 by Singing Dragon,
an imprint of Jessica Kingsley Publishers
An Hachette Company

1

Front cover image source: Daniel Hahn photographer and Christa Fairbrother model

A CIP catalogue record for this title is available from the
British Library and the Library of Congress

ISBN 978 1 83997 285 0
eISBN 978 1 83997 286 7

Printed and bound in the United States by Integrated Books International

Jessica Kingsley Publishers' policy is to use papers that are natural, renewable and recyclable
products and made from wood grown in sustainable forests. The logging and manufacturing
processes are expected to conform to the environmental regulations of the country of origin.

Jessica Kingsley Publishers
Carmelite House
50 Victoria Embankment
London EC4Y 0DZ

www.singingdragon.com

To all my teachers who have passed on their wisdom.

To my kids who keep stretching me.

*To my husband. Every mermaid needs a
rock for respite. You are my rock.*

Contents

Foreword

Want to make a difference? This book will lead you in helping yourself and helping others.

As the founder of the Aquatic Exercise Association and the Aquatic Therapy and Rehabilitation Institute, I'm completely behind the concept of better health through aquatics. Aquatics is the way to feel better, get fit, maintain function, and be happy. Whether through fitness or therapeutic formats, Christa has helped thousands of people improve their lives through time in the pool. Because of people like you and Christa, the benefits of aquatics have rippled out worldwide. *Water Yoga: A Teacher's Guide to Improving Movement, Health, and Wellbeing* further expands the rising tide of aquatics by enabling all of us in related disciplines to increase our skillsets and find alternative ways to teach in the pool.

Water yoga has so many varied applications. It can help regular people through exercise. Athletes can use it to advance training goals, or add it to therapeutic or rehabilitative movement programs. Finally, it can be used as a mind-body discipline to reduce stress. Until now, we've lacked a comprehensive guide for professionals to learn and apply water yoga.

Whether you are an aqua aerobics instructor, aquatic therapist, aquatic personal trainer, or land yoga instructor, who wants to teach water yoga or incorporate the tools of water yoga into what you already do, this book will guide you on that path. Get in the pool and learn this new material. Teach water yoga or use its principles to enhance the benefits of aquatics for your clients.

I've been impressed by Christa's ability to blend the diverse fields that water yoga represents. She incorporates aquatics, the sciences, and yoga in accessible language for various audiences, from yoga instructors, therapists, and personal trainers, to aquatics professionals looking to incorporate a more holistic mind-body experience for their clients. Christa presents material in a way that's actionable, evidence-based, and, most importantly, engaging. She is an outstanding instructor; she's articulate and good at both explaining concepts and applying them to real life.

Please remember to feed yourself first. As you read, focus on what this means to you and how you'd apply the ideas to yourself. Your body will thank you. You are better at sharing when you're healthy and have personally experienced the benefits. Then, after you've been using water yoga with others, come back to this book and review one chapter to refresh and refuel yourself. Your clients will thank you, and your entire community will benefit.

Water yoga is a coming trend. This book will prepare you to help others while you help yourself—physically, mentally, and emotionally. Enjoy this book, Christa's ideas, and making the world a better place.

Ruth Sova

Preface

Becoming a water yoga teacher is helping people embark on their journey into the sea of water yoga. Your students will use water yoga to reach their destination, whether it be a life with less pain, better balance, or less stress. They have a goal they want to achieve. No one sets off on an ocean voyage without some sort of boat. A person could get lost in all the waves. Your job is to help your students build the vessel that will ferry them to their destination. You can't build the boat for them, any more than you can do the yoga for them. You need to give them the tools and resources to create the container that's going to best serve them on their journey.

As such, becoming a water yoga teacher is like becoming the dean of a naval academy with a staff of one. You are now an instructor of boat-building, sail-making, celestial navigation, oceanography, and leadership. You need all the skills of a regular yoga teacher plus knowledge of the element of water. You're trying to help your students become effective captains of their own vessels through water yoga, the same way land-based yoga teachers or aquatics professionals are trying to build the agency and ownership of their practice within their students.

Trust is a background theme that runs throughout this book. You're placing your trust in me by reading this book and beginning your water yoga teaching journey. In turn, your students will put their trust in you as you guide them through these practices. Ultimately, your students will build trust in themselves by applying these principles. Everyone involved in this process is placing their trust in the healing, buoyant properties of water.

A part of building trust is being transparent and authentic. Knowing the story of the people you put your trust in is a window into their thought processes and perspective. My water yoga story might seem totally disjunct and random to some. However, all the various parts really do come together like high mountain runoff that percolates on its descent into one distinct waterfall.

I didn't know it at the time, but my water yoga journey began when I was 12 and my family took up skiing. While it was a blast, I'd swell up and turn red from the cold. It wasn't until I was around 18 that it became apparent there was a real pattern, and I saw a professional. The doctor suggested a rheumatoid arthritis test, which was negative, and so it just became a quirk that I was "allergic" to the cold.

After college, I became a farrier. It's not a job that's good for your back, but I'd heard somewhere that yoga was. I started attending an Iyengar yoga class with the attitude that it was preventative medicine. After several years, I found I really enjoyed yoga and how it made me feel. I developed a home practice that would get me warmed up for my days of cold barns and horse wrestling. I even appreciated how a yoga meditation was so similar to the peaceful repetitiveness of swimming laps in the pool. Those were my first baby steps toward becoming a yoga professional.

I continued to practice yoga through graduate school, and a career change into education. After the birth of my second son, my health took a turn for the worse. Yes, I now had two young kids, but that didn't explain being so tired that I was a hazard when driving. I did very little yoga that year. That's when I began making the rounds of the specialists who diagnosed me with systemic lupus erythematosus, an autoimmune disease.

Despite the health challenges, once both my kids started school, I decided it was time to enroll in yoga teacher training. Yoga had been such a constant in my life for 20 years. I didn't know if I wanted to teach, but I thought it would be a great opportunity to deepen my own practice. Almost halfway through my yoga teacher training, I got a new diagnosis: mixed connective disease, a combination connective tissue disease that is rare. I had been feeling happy I'd been doing a lot more yoga and hadn't had a lupus flare-up, but in reality, I'd had arthritis and lupus since I was a kid.

Getting that news was a blow. On the one hand, it made more sense with my symptoms over the years; on the other hand, it was tough to conceptually mesh my abilities with my diagnosis and imaging. How had I wrestled horses, pounded iron, and bucked hay for years while my body was destroying itself? Working out those discrepancies for myself made me decide to teach yoga at the end of the training. Years ago, I had stumbled on one of the best self-management tools I could have, and it had stuck. If I had benefited so much, I could help others stay pain free. I prioritized yoga trainings towards that goal and it was the water yoga that really resonated in the end.

On a personal level, adding the element of water took all the struggle out of a physical yoga practice, without taking anything away from all the other parts of yoga. In Ayurveda, the sister science of yoga, arthritis is considered a disease of drying out. Once I had that diagnosis, it made sense that I would love taking my yoga practice into the pool. I'd been a recreational swimmer even longer than I'd been a yogi. Water yoga allowed me to share what I was most passionate about in a way that benefited my health. It also professionally brought me full circle into why I loved shoeing horses.

As a farrier, I had the opportunity to work on horses that were in pain and struggling. They would limp up, obviously uncomfortable, and I had an hour to work my magic on them. The most satisfying part of the job was to watch that first step away from you of a horse you knew you'd helped. They expected to be in pain, and that first step would be in the same old movement pattern. But the limp was gone, and you could visibly see their bodies perk up with the relief. They walked away sound and happy, with the resounding clip-clop of a healthy horse. I relished the sense of satisfaction from a job well done.

The reason I love teaching water yoga isn't really any different. The timeframe is usually longer, but it's the reward of the positive feedback I get from my clients that pays off. One memorable client had been a shoe buyer for Macy's in New York City before she retired. She obviously loved stylish shoes and liked to joke that Imelda Marcos had learned her ways from her. When I started working with her, she only wore sensible walking shoes and used a cane. She had tripped one day and broken a hip. That accident, and the long recovery, had aggravated her ankle arthritis enough that she had had to have a joint replacement in her ankle. But that surgery had failed, and had to be done a second time. It still wasn't right, but she wasn't chancing a third time and had accepted that this was how her life was now.

She started coming to water yoga classes twice a week because she was intrigued by the title. She liked gentle aquatics classes and had never done yoga, but was curious. After coming to class for a couple months, she reduced how much time she used her cane. She only used it when she was worried about her footing, like on rainy days. More importantly to her, she felt so much more stable that she started wearing sandals again. After she had lunch with a friend one day, she broke down crying when she told me about it. For her lunch date, she had worn sandals and gone totally without her cane. She hadn't thought she would ever be able to do that again, and it meant the world to her. She told me I had made a beautiful difference in her life.

Keeping people out of pain and improving their lives in real tangible ways is why I love teaching water yoga. The forgiving, healing element of water allows me to reach people who can't attend regular yoga classes because of physical limitations. If you can't get on and off the ground, you don't have much use for mat yoga. Helping people who otherwise can't do yoga to improve their lives, in the ways that matter to them, is my water yoga "why." Water yoga will bring benefits to you through a personal practice, improve your students' lives, and impact your community in a way that will become your water yoga "why."

I appreciate the trust you've placed in me as an author, the trust you're showing in yourself to try new things, and the bravery you're showing in asking others to trust you. Trust in the water yoga journey.

Christa

Introduction

When you were little, did you daydream about being a mermaid? You rode your seahorse on fun adventures filled with color and friends. You were laughing and beautiful.

Or maybe you went to sea as the captain of a fast schooner. You always made the right decisions in tough situations. You were courageous and people counted on you.

Being a scallywag of a pirate might have been your thrilling escape. You led daring raids and your crew respected you. You were fun and strong.

Daydreaming about watery adventures isn't just for kids. Poets, authors, and storytellers of all stripes use the sea as the inspiration and setting for their tales because the sea captivates us. It's a blank slate we can project our desires onto. Our fantasies are out there if we can just reach out to the sunset and pluck them off the hazy horizon where the land and sea meet. We can daydream about the next amazing thing that's just beyond the horizon.

The ocean lets you find yourself, with just enough variety to keep it interesting. A mountain view can be beautiful, but it's fairly consistent and solid. It shows its changeability with the seasons, not in the moment. The sea is infinitely variable. Every wave, gust of wind, cloud pattern, and angle of the sun adds depth for your focus. Within its variety it is immutably strong. The sea is a force of nature. You can't hold back the waves any more than you can live underwater. We admire its power and changing moods and lose ourselves in it. It allows us to search for ourselves. We use phrases like, "sea of possibilities" or "sea of dreams."

Why do we care about being around the ocean and getting in the water? Everyone knows we need water for life. Go without a drink for several hours and your body will remind you of the necessity of it. But there's no biological need to go to the beach, and beach-front properties are always in more demand than inland locations.

A swimming pool allows us to bottle and contain the force of nature that is the sea. It brings the ocean into our backyards without the gritty sand or danger. We can splash and enjoy ourselves while controlling the temperature. We can swim till we get tired but never worry about getting swept out to sea. The deep end gives us a good workout without the threat of danger or death from sea creatures.

The safe, controlled environment of a swimming pool that can be thousands of miles inland allows people to benefit from being in the water, learn to swim, and engage in aquatic sports. It isn't just bringing poetry indoors, it's a practical venue that makes water activities, like water yoga, accessible to millions more people.

What exactly is water yoga? Basically, water yoga is taking all parts of yoga and practicing them in the water.

While that sounds like just a simple substitution, the change in environment produces profound differences in the practice. Water yoga is a combined discipline that takes the full spectrum of a yoga practice and submerges it. By engaging in yoga in the water, certain elements of the practice naturally rise to the surface and others fall by the wayside. Which elements those are will probably be a reflection of you, your history with aquatics, and your approach to yoga.

If you're an aqua aerobics professional, you already understand the profound benefits you can achieve by being in the water. You don't need to be convinced about the power of aquatics, you just need a nudge to help understand that being in the water doesn't have to be about how fast you can go or your cardio output. Water yoga can be a modality for helping people reach new goals, such as reducing stress and increasing their flexibility, as well as a sustainable way to extend your career as an aquatics professional by getting the benefits of practicing water yoga and teaching a slower-paced discipline that's not as hard on your body.

For aquatic therapists or anyone who uses the water therapeutically such as Watsu and Ai Chi professionals or aquatic physical therapists, water yoga can be a bridge for getting people to do their homework. There's more awareness about yoga as a discipline than aquatic therapy. Assigning yoga poses students can do between sessions might make them less hesitant to try the new work they're doing with you. Or they might have a friend who has more experience with yoga than they do. That person can provide some social support while they implement these techniques into their homework. Once they've created some personal aquatic habits, they're more likely to continue working both with you and independently, to gain long-term therapeutic benefits.

Swim coaches work with such a diversity of students, and water yoga can be another highly adaptable tool. Athletic swimmers can use water yoga to gain both flexibility and focus without having to leave the pool. Fearful new swimmers can improve their comfort level in the water and explore water movement in new ways as they build the confidence to get their hair wet. When working with kids, it's always challenging to keep them on task and engaged, so water yoga can be another fun way to keep them focused.

Both aquatics pros and yoga instructors bring something distinct to the field of water yoga. As you picked up this book, you have an interest in the subject, but are you coming to water yoga from an aquatics or a yoga background? If you've taught aqua aerobics or swim lessons, you have a lot of comfort with the water and understand how its properties affect bodies. If you've taught yoga, you understand yoga forms and philosophy. Each side is bringing half the equation to the table. This book bridges the gap for you. It teaches you how to present water yoga to your students in a way that allows them to receive the full benefits of the practice.

In my experience, yoga professionals are more hesitant to try yoga in the water. Some see it as a fad like goat yoga, or feel that it's just not real yoga since it's not on a mat. I think that attitude actually short-changes yoga since it implies that yoga isn't resilient or broad enough in its scope to still be yoga in a new environment. What this book shows is actually the opposite. Yoga is more than broad enough to encompass water yoga. Water yoga takes the practice and amplifies certain aspects to sharpen your skills. It brings a whole new level of accessibility to people who otherwise couldn't practice land yoga, and it opens up new possibilities within the scope of practice with the medium of water.

You might not be a pro at all, and are just curious about water yoga. There is a lack of resources and practice guides for this unique discipline so absolutely use these materials for yourself. Notice the teaching tips. Professionals are trained to help with the most common problems people face. If you try these techniques as a regular person without yoga experience and you struggle, the odds are that someone else does too and the solution is in this book. The do-it-yourself ethos is built into the discipline of yoga so you can be your own teacher with this book.

Thales, the ancient Greek who is considered the first philosopher, is credited with saying, "Everything is water," and that applies to yoga too.

— Chapter 1 —

Grounding Water Yoga

Yoga as a discipline was created over two thousand years ago in India. It seeks to harmonize the body, mind, and spirit to increase a person's wellbeing. The Sanskrit word yoga means to yoke, so it's seeking to unite a person's inner and outer worlds. It's an ancient tradition to understand the human condition which we all still face. As long as there are people, we will have to decide how we choose to live our lives, and that's why yoga continues to endure.

All types of yoga are grounded in the foundational texts of yoga, especially the sutras written by Patanjali. The sutras lay out yoga as a complete person practice made up of eight guiding principles or limbs. Each limb addresses one part of how yoga integrates your body, mind, and spirit. The limbs are a metaphor that ground your yoga practice and give it structure.

Metaphors give meaning to abstract concepts. However, for a water yoga practice, I think the metaphor of waves is more apt than limbs. Trees don't grow in the water and their rigidity doesn't make for effective symbolism in water yoga. The water is the essential element of a water yoga practice. Water yoga isn't just yoga in the pool. It's using the water to influence and expand the possibilities of yoga and what you can do with it.

If we are at the beach, the waves will continually lap at the shore. That unrelenting wave action serves as a valuable teaching example. The waves don't stop, so neither should your yoga practice. Every moment is a yoga moment, just as the sand is constantly interacting with the waves. Notice that there is no order to the waves at the beach. There is no first wave or last wave. That reinforces the idea of being able to practice the waves of water yoga in any order.

Some of these water yoga ideas will resonate with you more strongly than others. Start with the ideas you find easy and then begin to challenge yourself. Just as you wouldn't have a student dive into the deep end of a pool when they can't swim, don't start with the concepts you find overwhelming. Meet yourself where you are and then begin to dive a little deeper. Present the information to your students in the same metered way.

Most people know yoga because of the poses. However, yoga has not survived and prospered for thousands of years because of any particular exercise. A lunge in a yoga class is not a physically different shape than a lunge in a CrossFit gym. What is dramatically different is the attitude yoga brings to movement compared to other disciplines. That's because yoga isn't just about the physical body. The movements are meant to prepare your body to be better integrated with the mental, emotional, and spiritual aspects of yourself. As such, the eight waves address a diversity of ways we can integrate all parts of ourselves.

These are the eight waves of water yoga:

- Yamas: concepts you want to reduce in your life to treat yourself better.
- Niyamas: precepts you want to do more of to relate to other people better.
- Asanas: the movements we do in water yoga.
- Pranayama: breathwork.
- Pratyahara: focusing on yourself more, and what's going on around you less.
- Dharana: tools to improve your concentration during water yoga and the rest of your life.
- Dhyana: floating meditation.
- Samadhi: how to integrate all aspects of water yoga to be your best self.

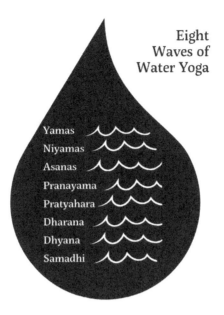

Eight
Waves of
Water Yoga

Yamas
Niyamas
Asanas
Pranayama
Pratyahara
Dharana
Dhyana
Samadhi

Water yoga frequently asked questions

You might already have these questions about water yoga, but these are the most common questions you'll get from the public.

Do you have to know how to swim to do water yoga?
No. You don't have to know how to swim because you don't have to submerge your face or head in water yoga. It helps if you're comfortable in the water because you're more relaxed but if this is your first time venturing into the pool, welcome.

Do you have to get your hair wet?
No. You keep your head above the surface of the water and you're welcome to wear a swim cap if you want to keep your hair dry.

Where do you practice water yoga?
The best place to practice water yoga is in a swimming pool because it's the most reliable. Using a therapy pool, hot tub, or lake, also works, but each has considerations that are covered in Chapter 14 on safety.

If you're lucky enough to have access to pleasantly warm ocean water, you can do water yoga in the sea. I've worked with teachers who teach in Mauritius in the Indian Ocean. They share beautiful pictures of their classes.

Where should you practice in the pool?

Ideally, you should be on a level surface submerged to mid-chest height, the height of your nipples. At that height, you reduce your weight-bearing by 75 percent. If you're in a shallower pool, it still works, and you offload 50 percent of weight at belly button height. Submerging up to your neck, you offload 90 percent of your weight, and you'll be too unstable to practice.

I've never done yoga before. Is that okay?

Absolutely. Water yoga makes a great introduction to yoga and, if you decide you want to, you can always add a land yoga practice to your yoga journeys.

What's water yoga good for?

Many people come to water yoga for a stretch and for better balance. However, water yoga is a full-person practice so you can also reduce your stress, get to know yourself better, and have a good time.

Who is water yoga for?

Just like land yoga, water yoga is for everyone. However, just like land yoga, there are many opportunities to focus on certain aspects of the practice and customize it for the individual.

Everything about yoga is designed to increase the agency of you, the participant, in all aspects of your life. To that end the eight waves of water yoga are practical, applicable concepts to help you live your best life, not just enjoy your time in the pool.

— Chapter 2 —

Incorporating Yoga Philosophy during Water Yoga

The Yamas and Niyamas represent the first and second waves of water yoga respectively. Yoga philosophy is the foundation of what makes yoga, yoga, and not just random movement. Keeping every aspect of water yoga informed by the Yamas and Niyamas is what distinguishes it from other forms of aquatic exercise. It's vital as a teacher that you have a working knowledge of yoga philosophy to present the discipline as a complete practice.

These are my definitions of the ten Yamas and Niyamas. I have kept the original intent but rephrased the translations to be positive actions. The first Yama, Ahimsa, is traditionally translated as non-harming. I'm a parent of two boys. If I tell one of my boys, "Don't hit your brother," what happens? One brother gets hit. If instead, I say, "Use loving touch only," I'm more likely to get the kind of interaction I'm looking for between my kids. I've done the same thing with these translations.

The Yamas are traditionally restraints, and ways to reduce certain behaviors in ourselves. I've turned them around to be things we want to do more of for ourselves. That's also more in line with the Niyamas, which are traditionally positive ways we can relate to others.

A water yoga perspective on the five Yamas
Ahimsa: Being kind

Practicing Ahimsa is about being kind to yourself and others. You can think of Ahimsa as the integration of all aspects of a well-built harbour, which protects the water quality of its local ecosystem, provides safe haven for the boats that dock there, and is a good neighbor in its community. Applying the metaphor of what makes a good harbor to your water yoga practice, you can learn to take care of yourself, be kind to others, and still have good boundaries.

As teachers, we often struggle with Ahimsa by demoing postures too deeply, or too often, and hurt ourselves. Your students will push themselves in poses as well. Ahimsa moves water yoga from "No pain, no gain" to "No pain, no pain."

Satya: Being truthful

You always listen to the lifeguard on the pool deck because they give you directions geared towards keeping you and everyone else safe. They speak with honesty and integrity. Satya is about developing an inner lifeguard to guide you, an inner voice that will help you stay in your lane.

As a teacher, you can run into trouble by not staying in your scope of practice. You need to be honest about your qualifications and skills. Conversely, you need your students to be honest with their health status. Often in public classes, you'll have no information about your students and be hampered in your ability to help them effectively. Satya is aiming for an honest exchange of information and energy.

Asteya: Being generous

Jules Verne's *20,000 Leagues under the Sea* could be considered one of the first books to call for ocean conservation. It pits the idea of taking whatever you want from the ocean at any cost, against the wisdom of being a good steward of natural resources. Asteya helps us distinguish between what's mine, what's yours, and what's ours effectively.

Be generous with your knowledge and time with your students and colleagues. Sharing freely does not exclude you from being fairly compensated. Your students need to share the pool and gear with everyone else who's there. Hoarding is not good stewardship. Practicing water yoga with the humility to recognize that yoga is not a finite resource allows you to be generous and share time, space, and knowledge with others.

Brahmacharya: Using your energy wisely

Long-distance swimmers have to learn to conserve their energy so that they can finish crossing the English Channel or whatever race they're in. Practicing Brahmacharya is learning how to pace yourself to always have the energy for the task at hand.

A cat never misses a cat nap to go to work, but we as teachers will do that, and our students will make poor choices that overtax their energy. Brahmacharya teaches us that water yoga should revitalize us, not become something else to do as a burden, or something that we regret later.

Aparigraha: Being grateful

The antidote to greed and grasping is gratitude and openness. Practicing with an expansive attitude of gratitude will bring you more happiness than a narrow focus on scarcity.

Water yoga is a perfect Aparigraha practice for yoga teachers because learning the techniques and how to teach them requires us to become open to new yoga ideas and approaches to teaching. You have to soften your grip on old ideas and welcome new knowledge. Students will often express regret or surprise about how hard water yoga is and be disappointed they didn't do better. No one is perfect at anything the first time, and their disappointment is often driven by their expectations. Aparigraha teaches us to be grateful for opportunities for growth, instead of regret for the things that no longer serve us.

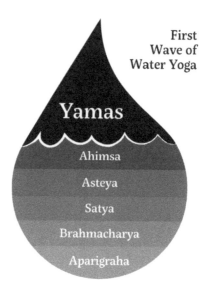

First
Wave of
Water Yoga

Yamas

Ahimsa

Asteya

Satya

Brahmacharya

Aparigraha

A water yoga perspective on the five Niyamas
Saucha: Taking care of yourself

Saucha is the water yoga equivalent of "Mermaid hair, don't care" that you see on beach T-shirts. It's a path to a better body image and positive self-talk because it gives you tools to overcome vanity and internalized shame. With Saucha, you are unapologetically taking care of yourself.

Wearing whatever outfit you need to on the pool deck, teaching while in the water, and taking a water break while teaching are all examples of practicing Saucha as a teacher. Encourage your students to do the same. Make your water yoga classes a place of radical self-care.

Santosha: Contentment

Contentment is a deeper level of satisfaction than fleeting happiness. If you can stay focused on your own internal motivation instead of external rewards, you can develop an attitude of equanimity. When you go fishing, there's no guarantee you're going to catch anything. That's why it's called fishing and not catching. When you stay focused on why you went fishing, and how much you enjoy spending time outside by the water, it doesn't matter if you catch fish or not.

As a teacher, you'll make mistakes when you teach; you'll misspeak, mirror incorrectly, and forget cues. That doesn't mean you offered a bad class. The same thing applies to your students. They might struggle in one pose one day, but that doesn't mean they can't enjoy water yoga ever again. Santosha is about perspective and focusing on the bigger picture.

Tapas: Do your best

Instead of lurching between the poles of an extreme sports approach to movement and a barnacle that never leaves its rock, Tapas encourages just the right amount of effort. If you're phoning it in, you're not disappointing anyone else. You're only cheating yourself. If you hurt after your practice, you're the one paying the price. Tapas teaches you how to find the middle ground that represents your personal best.

For teachers, Tapas means we present ourselves professionally while maintaining a good work–life balance. Some teachers will push themselves and try and teach five classes a day, five days a week and demonstrate every move. Others will teach the same class every session for years. Tapas means you're dedicated to your craft as a professional while not losing sight of the other Yamas and Niyamas. You'll see your students struggle with being Type A and always pushing, or not paying attention and trying to chat through the class. Be a Tapas role model by applying the right effort.

Svadhyaya: Self-knowledge

Practicing Svadhyaya transforms you into an explorer of your inner depths like Jacques Cousteau venturing undersea. It's approaching water yoga as your own personal science experiment to create an evidence-informed practice that helps you learn about yourself. The same way you test and monitor the pH in your pool, you try out different water yoga techniques and assess what works for you, and what doesn't.

Because we are all individuals, it's important that you're clear on your approach to your personal practice versus your teaching philosophy so that you can differentiate between the two in the best interests of your students. Your classes are about your students, not you.

Increasing their self-knowledge is one of the most powerful things your students will gain from their water yoga practice. Svadhyaya is an important baseline skill to ensure that you apply the right tools of water yoga at the right time, and in the right amount.

Ishvara Pranidhana: Trust your inner guidance

The North Star is a traditional navigation point for mariners because of its stable position in the night sky. You can use it on your water yoga adventures too. Let your intuition and inner guidance become your North Star navigation point. Your internal reference points are more relevant than anyone else's opinion. Use all the Yamas and Niyamas together to create your own wayfinding chart to guide you in the direction you need to go on your water yoga travels.

Teachers will sometimes struggle with Ishvara Pranidhana because they lack the confidence to share yoga philosophy. You might think people won't be interested or only want a workout. Some students have heard yoga is a religion and this Niyama becomes a barrier for them to practice at all. Ishvara Pranidhana simply integrates all the aspects of yoga philosophy to connect you with yourself so that your water yoga practice serves and honors you.

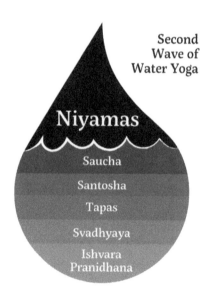

Teaching tips for sharing water yoga philosophy with your students

- Use a translation of the yoga sutras that resonates with you, and that you understand as a reference.
- Meet people where they are. Some students will be more interested than others, and that's okay.
- Respect the venue where you're teaching. Some venues may be more accepting of yoga philosophy than others.
- Focus on one concept at a time, and incorporate the same concept several times during a session.
- Try to make yoga philosophy relevant to both your students' water yoga practice and their daily lives.
- Share yoga philosophy during the session when people can hear easily.
- Honor the Sanskrit but always use English language translations also.
- Repetition helps students. Don't feel as if you have to share new concepts every time.

Applied teaching examples

Pick one yoga sutra that resonates with you. Introduce the sutra at the beginning of class as the theme for the day. Repeat the sutra with two relevant poses. Share the sutra again before meditating.

For example, I share sutra 3.25 as:

By directing your perception, you gain awareness of subtle, hidden, and remote parts of yourself. Today, we're going to practice by really digging deep into the subtle aspects of what's going on within ourselves. I encourage you to pay attention to things you wouldn't necessarily notice while you practice, like do you have as much weight on your left pinky toe as your right as you move through the poses? Or is the length of your inhale and exhale the same in all your postures?

Be open to what else you'll notice when you get in touch with these tiny details.

Repeat the sutra and its ideas, with different prompts that support the concepts you're trying to get across, throughout the session.

Another example would be to choose a Yama or Niyama that resonates with you. Challenge students to keep their practice aligned with the ideas of that Yama or Niyama.

For example, if you choose Ahimsa, explain it means non-harming, and challenge people to keep their practice kind. When doing an easy posture like Standing Twist, ask people to check in with themselves physically and energetically. Can they identify what being kind to themselves looks like in this posture? When doing a challenging posture like Dancer's pose, can they still practice Ahimsa? Would applying Ahimsa during Dancer's pose mean doing a variation, using a prop, changing the length of the hold of the pose? Before they meditate, ask them to think about how they can apply this idea outside the pool, perhaps examining how they talk to themselves, or identifying something that physically annoys them like a poorly fitting office chair. Bring it back around to Ahimsa during meditation by inviting them to choose the most comfortable floating position. Remind them there are no mistakes during meditation; there are only opportunities to practice again.

Yoga philosophy can be a dedicated area of study on its own, as well as a lifelong learning journey. This is an introduction to the area that will serve you in your water yoga teaching needs. As you continue to dive deeper into the practice, there are specialists in yoga philosophy that you can learn from and adapt to yoga in the pool.

— Chapter 3 —

Using Water Yoga Props

We use props, tools, equipment, and gear in water yoga for similar reasons as we would use them in land yoga or aqua aerobics classes—they help us in our practice. They provide support, challenge us, increase variety, and teach us about how we use our bodies. The three most common props in water yoga are pool noodles, aquatic dumbbells, and kickboards.

Here are some general points about water yoga props:

- Always inspect your props to ensure they're in good working order before handing them out.
- The most common water yoga props are buoyant equipment made of plastic or foam. They naturally float and require muscular effort to move through the water.
- Match the prop to the person using it. For example, a person who's a "sinker" will need more buoyant equipment than a naturally floaty person.
- All movements with props are easier closer to the torso as short lever movements, and harder when further away as long lever ones (see Chapter 12 for more information on levers).
- Buoyant props allow you to both change the water depth you work at and suspend your feet off the pool floor. In aquatics, a level one movement would be a water yoga pose with your feet attached to the pool floor like Chair pose. The majority of water yoga poses are level one movements. Level two movements have

more of your body submerged, and your feet are sometimes off the pool floor. For example, use a prop alongside your body in Chair pose to bring your feet up off the pool floor. Straighten one leg in front and one leg behind you into the splits. By alternating which leg is attached to the pool floor in front and which is attached behind, with a floating Chair pose when you switch in the middle, you're doing a level two movement. If you stay fully suspended in your Chair pose, supporting yourself on each side of your body with a prop, you're in a level three movement. Level three movements are entirely off the pool floor and are less common in water yoga.

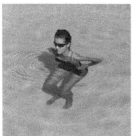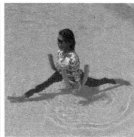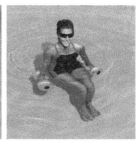

Level One, Two and Three Movements

- The surface tension of the water is more impactful when using props. People who have trouble with their shoulders will potentially struggle with moving a prop in and out of the water. Best practice is cueing for a prop to stay under, or above, the water's surface for anyone with shoulder challenges. You can also cue students to bring the prop to the surface as an intermediate step, rather than straight up and down. It slows the action, and allows people to prepare for surface tension, therefore it's less demanding. Consider this with Sun Salutations, or any standing poses where you'll raise and lower the arms.
- Make sure all props are cleaned and put away properly after using them.

Noodles

Pool noodles are your most versatile water yoga prop and are read-ily available. Noodles come in two chief styles: hollow or solid core. Also, there are usually two diameters to choose from: a smaller at approximately two and a quarter inches in diameter, or a larger that's approximately three and a quarter inches. You want noodles in the smaller diameter as they're more versatile. The ones they sell at the dollar store are fine. The pool noodles sold at pool supply stores are slightly better quality foam and are usually a bit more buoyant. They will also last longer. The solid core noodles are more buoyant than the hollow core ones.

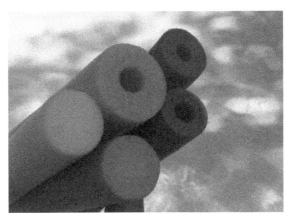

Examples of pool noodles

Ways to use pool noodles:

- As passive support, such as in a floating meditation.
- As buoyancy aids in active postures, such as Cobra pose.
- To challenge your strength and balance by using them under the water in your hands, such as Humble Warrior pose.
- Under your feet to increase your body awareness and balance, such as Warrior III pose.
- Tied in knots to mimic a dumbbell.

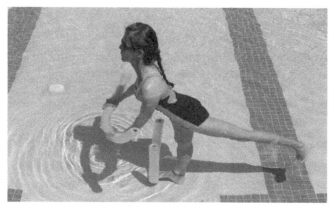

*Warrior III with a noodle under the standing
leg and underwater in the hands*

Dumbbells

Dumbbells come in a variety of styles and buoyancy levels. Provide comfortable dumbbells that have enough buoyancy to challenge students, without forcing them out of good form. Examples of this include using the dumbbells with the elbows out to the sides, or hiking the shoulders up.

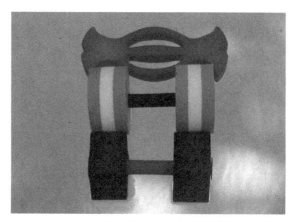

Example of aquatic dumbbells

Dumbbells can do most of the things noodles do with some key differences:

- Dumbbells offer the advantage of individualized hand movement (unlike one noodle), without the square footage requirements of two pool noodles.
- Dumbbells can aggravate people's hands and shoulders. They might grip the handles too tight or be using a dumbbell that's too buoyant for them. Build in breaks to let go of the prop and let students relax their hands. Provide alternatives such as noodles, no props, or the wall. Also, there are more therapeutic styles of dumbbells that are easier on the hands.

Kickboards

The kickboards you use in water yoga are the same kickboards swimmers use while swimming laps.

- Kickboards can be used through the water as a buoyant prop that offers a lot of resistance, on the water's surface to create stability, or under your bum as a floating seat.
- Don't try to stand on the kickboard. They are too buoyant and will come shooting out. They could hurt you or someone else.
- Because kickboards are so buoyant, they don't offer a lot of stability under the water. For that reason, they're more effective in active postures. Switch to other props during floating meditation.

Other props you can experiment with include yoga blocks, yoga belts, rubber resistance bands, weights, buoyancy cuffs, or drag equipment.

Muscular effort with water yoga props

Muscular effort is different in the water, so here's a quick review of muscular effort on land, compared to muscular effort in the water.

On land, muscular load against gravity's resistance (bending your elbow to bring your palm towards your shoulder) is a concentric contraction. A concentric contraction shortens your muscle, in this case, your biceps, as it responds to force. Muscular load with gravity (straightening your elbow to bring your hand back down against your body) is an eccentric contraction. An eccentric contraction makes your muscle lengthen in response to load. It decelerates joint movement and creates more force than a concentric contraction. You can grab your biceps with your other hand as you do this to feel the muscle move.

A third muscular action is an isometric contraction. There the muscle is concentrically contracted and then held. For example, an isometric contraction in your biceps happens in the middle of a Low Plank pose against the pool wall. Your biceps concentrically contract when you lower yourself down towards the pool edge. Your biceps isometrically contract to hold you in your Plank position while you're there. Your biceps eccentrically contract to push you back up to regular Plank pose. The action of an isometric contraction is the same on land or underwater because your muscle length doesn't change in response to force. Many traditional yoga poses on land or in the water use isometric contractions to build strength.

While moving through the water, muscular effort is different because of the water's viscosity. In the water without props, there is resistance from the water's viscosity in every direction. Therefore, every muscular contraction is a concentric contraction.

Muscular effort changes again when using a buoyant prop like dumbbells or noodles in the water because the prop changes the direction of effort your muscles are moving against. Instead of resisting the downwards pull of gravity, the direction of resistance is dictated by the prop.

Assisting buoyancy is using a buoyant prop underwater while your body moves with buoyancy towards the water's surface. This is usually described as feeling as if the muscular action is easier. If you hold a dumbbell in your hand and repeat your biceps curl, bringing your hand up to your shoulder is easier now because of the buoyancy of the dumbbell. When performing an action that assists buoyancy, the muscular effort is eccentric. Think about the effort you're exerting to control the speed of bending your elbow in this example.

Resisting buoyancy is using a buoyant prop underwater, while your body is resisting the prop popping up towards the surface of the water. This is usually described as making the muscular action feel harder. To straighten your arm down to your side after doing your biceps curl above, it's going to take a lot more effort when moving a buoyant dumbbell underwater. When performing an action that resists buoyancy, the muscular effort is concentric.

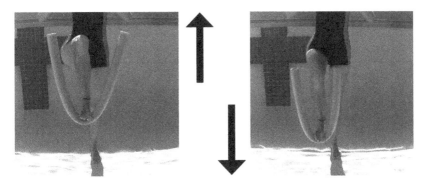

Assisting vs. resisting buoyancy

A buoyant prop basically reverses the muscular effort involved compared to on land. Knowing which muscular actions happen with each prop, and when, helps you give effective cues to your students, helps you answer their questions, and makes you a better teacher. As you practice, these actions will become more instinctual for you.

Using buoyancy to affect your body is only possible in the water. Props help you control and direct buoyancy's impacts in new and beneficial ways. Because the impact of buoyancy on your body is not instinctual, using props highlights the importance of having a personal water yoga practice as a teacher. Part of being a good teacher is communicating what people might feel and what problems they might have, before they occur, to increase student success. If you're not clear on how the various props act in all the different poses, you won't be able to share that. When learning all the poses in the next chapter, try each of them with all the different prop options. Get creative with the props and poses to be a great teacher.

— Chapter 4 —

Teaching Water Yoga Asanas

Asanas are the poses we do in water yoga. It's the third wave of water yoga. Even though it's not the first wave, it's the best-known segment of yoga and what students are most comfortable with. It can feel like a tsunami compared to the other waves of water yoga. Since the poses are why most people are coming to your classes, we cover the subject in depth. The other waves of water yoga work in tandem with the poses.

A note about the order of these postures. These postures are not arranged alphabetically. They're grouped into five sections based on how often you use them, and the ease of practicing them. This means you always do more standing postures than seated postures, so standing postures are first. The poses are laid out roughly from the easiest/most common to the hardest/less common, within each section. This makes it easier to put them together when we talk about sequencing later.

For ease of language, all the directions for poses are given to the right side. All poses should be done in both directions. When doing the left side, simply reverse the words.

In your Asana practice, you strive for balance. That means you want to practice each pose in each direction, but that doesn't necessarily mean that each posture looks exactly the same side to side. Offer the postures to your students in both directions. The students live in their own bodies. Encourage them to listen to their bodies. If they need to make adjustments on one side versus the other, they should act on that.

For example, shoulder injuries are commonly one-sided. A student might raise one arm up fully overhead on one side, while on the injured side, the hand only comes to the top of the head. Body awareness and good use of yoga philosophy always trumps cookie-cutter symmetry.

Each posture starts with the cueing directions for the base pose. Most of them also have variations that you can add in to maintain accessibility and variety for your students, as well as teaching tips that highlight the most common issues you'll see as a teacher. The English names come first, followed by the Sanskrit to honor the tradition of yoga.

Standing poses
Mountain pose or Tadasana

For Mountain pose, or Tadasana, your feet start hip-bone distance apart. Your feet are parallel. Most of us need to rotate our thighs inwards a little to make that happen. Heels pushing out is another way to think of it. Your knees and hips stack over your feet. Your front ribs draw back towards the spine, and your chest lifts. Your chin tucks in towards your throat to bring your ears over your shoulders and lengthen the back of your neck.

Without a prop, your arms are straight out of your shoulder sockets in a T-shape, palms facing down on the surface of the water to support you. If you press your palms against the surface of the water, as if it were a solid instead of a liquid, you will feel more attached to the pool floor. This is easier to do with the fingers spread. With a prop, press down on it slightly to engage your torso muscles. Breathe. Root down into the ground like a mountain.

Another option to increase your stability is to bring all ten toes up off the pool floor, root your feet, and set your toes back down.

VARIATIONS

- Raise your arms overhead for Extended Mountain (Utthita Tadasana). Look straight ahead or up at your raised hands.

- Do this with one or both hands on the pool wall for more support.
- Your back can be against the pool wall with your arms out to the sides on the pool deck for support and upper body lift.

TEACHING TIPS

- Most students set their feet too wide and turn their toes out.
- Some students hyperextend their knees.
- Encourage neutral spine instead of hyperlordosis or kyphosis.

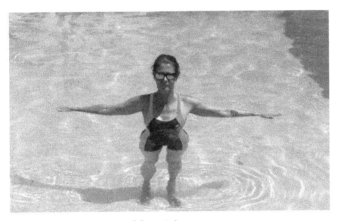

Mountain pose

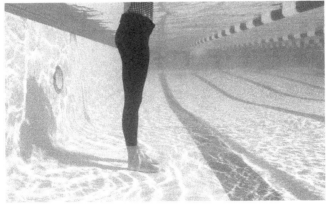

Mountain pose underwater from the side

Standing Twist or Parivrtta Tadasana

For Standing Twist pose, or Parivrtta Tadasana, start in Mountain pose with your hands on the surface of the water. Inhale, and on an exhale, open your right hand and the right side of your body to the right, allowing your spine to twist any amount. Inhale back to the center. Exhale and twist to the left. Your gaze can follow the hand that's opening up or look straight ahead. If you're using props, allow them to follow you around. Keep your feet in Mountain pose as you twist. Emphasize moving with your breath and finish back in Mountain pose.

VARIATIONS

- Add variation to a Standing Twist by changing the base, for example wide versus narrow, from the photos.
- Add variation by rotating only the torso rather than opening the arms.
- Depending on which prop you're using, cue for the appropriate upper body actions.

TEACHING TIPS

- Students will let their feet wiggle all over the place as they twist. Encourage staying in Mountain pose.
- Complaints about knee pain are usually about too much twist, which we're prone to do in the water. Encourage backing off a little.
- Students lead with their gaze and twist more in their neck than anywhere else. Introduce the concept of not overdriving your headlights. You don't move your head more than your headlights when you're driving in the car, so don't turn your neck more than your belly button.
- Cue the twist to be timed to your breath. Whipping side to side quickly is an indication of not moving with the breath.

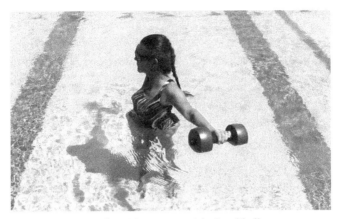

Standing Twist pose with dumbbells

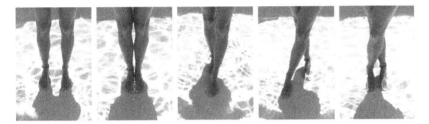

Foot position options for Standing Twists and Side Stretches

Side Stretch or Urdhva Hastasana

Side Stretch pose, or Urdhva Hastasana, can be done in many variations. These directions are for a wide-legged side stretch. From Mountain pose, step your feet out wide—wider than shoulder-distance. Keep
your feet parallel as if you were straddling railroad tracks. Bring your
arms straight out of your shoulder sockets in a T-shape, palms facing
up. At this point, you're in Five-Pointed Star pose. In your T, inhale.
As you exhale, bring your right arm up overhead and bring the left
arm down against your left thigh. Pretend you're sliding your thumbs
up and down along a wall behind you. That keeps your shoulders back
and stacked on top of your hips. Inhale back to a T and repeat to the
left on an exhale. Emphasize moving with your breath and finish in
Mountain pose in the center.

VARIATIONS

- Choose a foot position first: normal, wide, narrow, tandem, or crossed.
- Your hands can stay on your hips, or raise them to your shoulders, or the top of your head.
- With a buoyant prop, both your arms can stay under the water at your sides. Your arms remain straight, and your torso bends. You build strength by resisting the buoyant prop in your hands while getting a stretch too.

TEACHING TIPS

- Many students have shoulder injuries. Offer lots of arm variations or different options for each arm.
- Students tend to lean forward and bring their top shoulder and arms in front of their face. Encourage keeping the shoulders back in the same plane as the hips, and the hand behind the line of sight.
- When doing the variations that resist buoyancy, students want to bend their elbows. That's ungrounding and hard on their joints. Encourage straight arms and making this about movement in the torso.

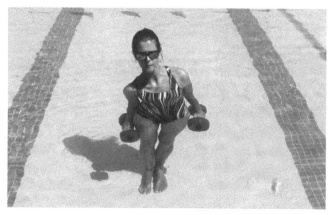

Side Stretch pose with dumbbells

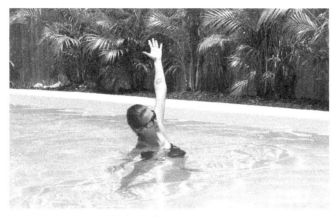

Wide-legged Side Stretch pose

Standing Half-Locust pose or Salabhasana

For Half-Locust pose, or Salabhasana, start in Mountain pose. Bend your right knee and extend the right leg behind you. Point your toes, and secure your right toes to the pool floor. Keep both your hips and shoulders parallel to the pool floor and facing forward instead of dropping down or twisting back to the extended foot. Inhale and raise your left arm up, then lower your left hand down. Then, leaving the legs where they are, try raising the right arm to work on the same side. See how that feels (most people find that harder). Step back up to Mountain pose with your right foot.

VARIATIONS

- If you follow the moving hand with your gaze, it increases the challenge.
- There are lots of possible arm combinations with or without a prop. Think about movement in all planes (not just sagittal, but transverse and coronal).
- You can also do a prone variation with a prop. Come to the tops of both the feet, as in Cobra pose. Add in lifting the legs one at a time instead of arm movement. This has more similarities to the traditional land-based prone Locust pose.

- Students often want to make extending the leg back a big step and then bend their knees. Emphasize that this is with straight legs, and your back leg is acting like a kickstand behind you.

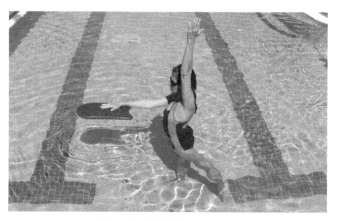

Standing Half-Locust pose

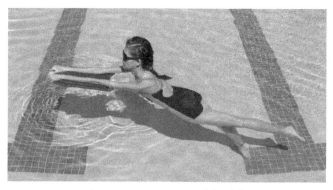

Prone Locust pose with leg lift

Pyramid pose or Parsvottonasana

For Pyramid pose, or Parsvottonasana, start in Mountain pose. Step forward with your right foot two steps. Your feet need to be parallel and both heels on the ground. If your left heel is rising up, or your left toes are turning out, the steps were too big, and you need to shorten your stance. If you want more stretch, inhale, and on exhale hinge forward with both hips keeping your spine straight and long. On an inhale, come back up to standing. Step back with your right foot to finish in Mountain pose.

VARIATIONS

- Your arms can be anywhere, but on your hips is easiest. Opening them out, bringing them behind your back, or raising them up is progressively harder.
- A prop can also go behind your back held with both hands to help you keep your spine straight.
- This also works well at the wall—either facing the wall with the hands on the pool deck, or with the back heel against the pool wall.
- For more stretch, raise all ten toes while you're in the posture.

TEACHING TIPS

- Students round their torsos forward and collapse their spines. Cue the hip hinge and emphasize keeping the chest lifted with a straight spine.
- Don't jut your chin forward. Cue keeping it tucked in towards the throat.
- Your feet stay parallel, and the back heel stays down.

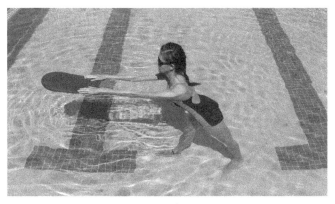

Pyramid pose

Chair pose or Utkatasana

For Chair pose, or Utkatasana, start in Mountain pose. Your arms can be anywhere. Inhale in the center. Exhale and bend your knees, sinking down into an imaginary chair. Look down at your knees. Are they close together? If that's the case, bring them back to hip bone distance apart and concentrate on weighting the outer edges of your feet. When you look down, have your feet turned out? If so, bring your feet back to parallel.

Concentrate on leaving your feet where you put them by weighting the outer edge. Where is your weight front to back? Are you back on your heels or up on your toes? Try to weight the center of your foot front to back and concentrate on being firm with the outer edge. If Chair pose challenges your low back, try tucking your pubic bone and tail bone towards your nose to create more length in your low back. Straighten your legs to come back into Mountain pose.

VARIATIONS

- Revolve your Chair pose to the side. Bring your hands to your heart, fingertips and palms touching with bent elbows. Inhale in the center. As you exhale, bring one elbow down towards your knees, twisting in your torso. Come back to the center and repeat to the other side.
- Add any arm position. Movement with the arms above, on the surface, or through the water are all options. Adding a prop to the hands expands the choices.
- Bring your Chair pose to the tiptoes.
- Straighten one leg out in front or behind you and add movement by sweeping the leg through the water.
- Lift one leg off the pool floor and add a balance challenge.
- Add a noodle under one or both feet. A noodle can also go behind the back of the thighs.

TEACHING TIPS

- Students almost always start too wide, shift their feet (usually out), and pivot their knees (often in) in Chair pose. Encourage keeping your feet and knees hip-bone distance apart. Increasing the weight on the outside edge of the feet can help.
- When revolving Chair pose, students will shift the knees. The knee in the direction they're turning towards will shift back. Encourage them to keep the knees from shifting. Using a trimmed pool noodle like a yoga block between the knees can help illuminate this point.
- Students often hold their breath in Chair pose. Encourage Ahimsa despite being fierce.

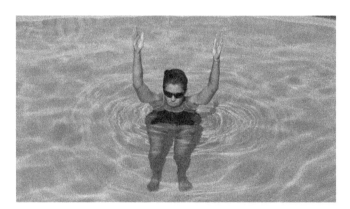

Chair pose

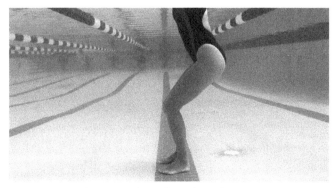

Chair pose from the side underwater

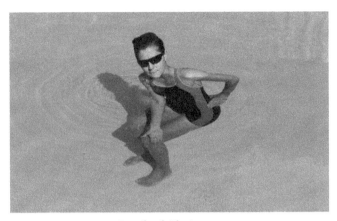

Revolved Chair pose

Cat/Cow pose or Marjariasana/Bitilasana

For Cat/Cow pose, or Marjariasana/Bitilasana, start in Chair pose. Inhale in the center. Exhale, bring your hands together in front of you as you round your spine away from your belly button, and look down towards the water. It's as if you've rounded into a snail shell. Inhale, bring your hands out to a T on the water's surface. Lift your chest, and maybe look up towards the sky. Exhale, back into a rounded spine. Keep your legs in your Chair pose as you move your spine and arms. Straighten the legs and come back up to Mountain pose when you're done.

VARIATIONS

- This can be done with any prop.
- When you bring your hands apart and lift your chest, straighten your legs back up to Mountain pose. When you exhale and round your spine, sink back down into your Chair pose.
- When you extend your spine and stand, step forward with one foot. Exhale and step back into Chair pose while rounding into the snail shell. Inhale, stand, and lift the chest while stepping forward with the other leg.

TEACHING TIPS

- Students tend to concentrate movement in their necks for this pose. Encourage equal movement in all three parts of their spine.

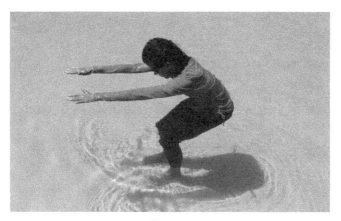

Cat pose

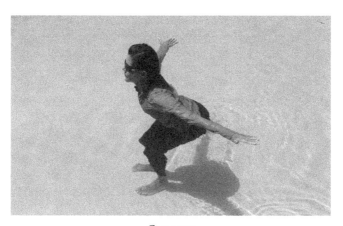

Cow pose

Down Dog pose or Adho Mukha Svanasana

For Down Dog pose, or Adho Mukha Svanasana, start in Mountain pose with one noodle under each of your armpits and your forearms resting on the noodles. Step wide with your feet, at least wider than shoulder-distance. Keep your feet parallel as if you are straddling railroad tracks, as in the Side Stretch. Your heels and bum are going to stay back on an imaginary wall. Inhale, and as you exhale, hinge forward in your hips. Keep your spine straight and your weight in your heels. Energetically draw your bum away from your hands into your imaginary wall. Inhale and come back up to wide-legged Mountain pose. Step, or heel-toe your feet back together to Mountain pose.

VARIATIONS

- Use any prop for this posture, or none at all.
- Try the pose with hands on the pool deck or your bum against the pool wall.

TEACHING TIPS

- The first time students do this, they usually fall forward no matter how often you say, "anchor through your heels" or, "weight the soles of your feet." It's okay, makes for a good laugh, and then try again.
- When using the noodles, shorter people need to drop their forearms inside the noodles so the noodles don't make their shoulders ride up.

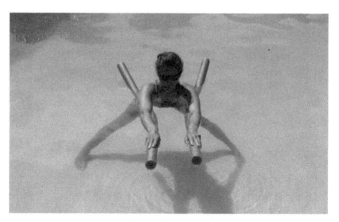

Down Dog pose

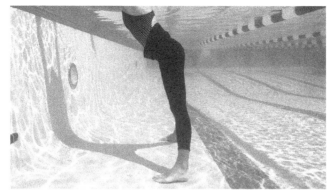

Down Dog pose using the pool wall underwater

Revolved Down Dog pose or Parivrtta Adho Mukha Svanasana

The last time you're in Down Dog pose, try revolving it. In your Down Dog, exhale and open one noodle out to the side. Inhale back to the center, and exhale and open the other noodle out to the side. Look straight ahead or back at the revolving noodle. Come back to wide-legged Mountain pose, then step, or heel-toe your feet back together to Mountain pose.

VARIATIONS

- Instead of opening one arm at a time in an open twist, keep both arms parallel while you twist.
- This can be done with or without props.
- Try the pose with the hands on the pool deck, or the bum against the wall.

TEACHING TIPS

- I usually teach this in three rounds. As students rotate around each time, they get a little more upright, so by the time they've done it three times, they're standing upright instead of hinged forward in Down Dog pose. Because it happens virtually every time, I include this habit in my directions and cue people to stay in their Down Dog pose as they revolve it.

- This is an excellent pose for swimming teachers to teach the torso roll required for early swimming skills, without a student having to get their hair wet.

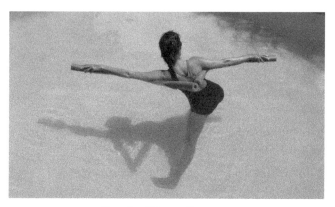

Revolved Down Dog pose

Triangle pose or Trikonasana

For Triangle pose, or Trikonasana, take a wide-legged stance, wider than shoulder-distance, with parallel feet. Turn your right toes out 90 degrees, turn your left toes in towards the right a hair more. Your arms come straight out of your shoulders, approximately wrists above ankles. Pretend you've got an imaginary wall behind you that your back body is touching. As you exhale, hinge in your right hip and allow your right hand to slide along your imaginary wall. When you have no more hinge in your hip, you stop. The left arm can stay on the surface of the water, come to your waist, or raise up perpendicularly. To come out, lower the left arm and bring your torso back to upright. Step or heel-toe your feet back together to Mountain pose.

VARIATIONS

- The top arm can be anywhere. Think about movement opportunities in the transverse and coronal planes.

- Raising the toes on the leading foot, putting the leading foot toes on a noodle, or on a step, will increase the challenge.

TEACHING TIPS

- Any distance between the feet, as long as it's at least shoulder width, is fine.
- Your leading hip, knee, and toes should all be pointing the same direction.
- Look for students turning the back toes out rather than straight ahead, or in towards the leading toes.
- Students will drop the top hip forward towards the pool floor, instead of stacking it on top of the lower. The top shoulder will then roll forward also.
- Help students protect their top shoulder. The top arm should raise only if they can keep the shoulder back. The top arm does not need to raise; it can come to the waist, or the shoulder.
- It's called Triangle pose because your legs make a triangle shape. People will often bend the front knee, so use the name to reiterate that point. Don't be a quadrilateral!

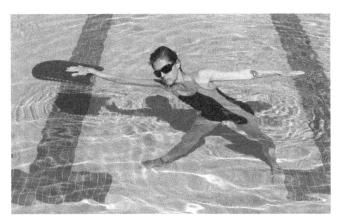

Triangle pose with a kickboard

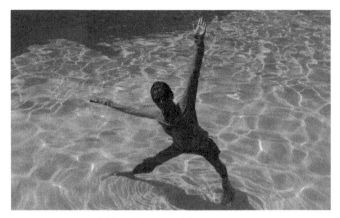

Triangle pose without props

Revolved Triangle pose or Parivrtta Trikonasana

For Revolved Triangle pose, or Parivrtta Trikonasana, set yourself up like starting Triangle pose to the right side. Turn your hips to face your right toes and bring your arms perpendicular to your feet. Your belly button and your shoulders are now facing the same direction as your right toes. Your left toes might need to point towards the right toes more. Turn your shoulders to bring the left hand towards your right foot. Hinge forward with both hips. Reach the right hip back and the left hip forward by energetically bringing your feet closer together even though they are not moving on the pool floor. Your left arm stays on the surface of the water. Your right hand can be on the surface of the water, at your waist, or raised up. Unwind back to Five-Pointed Star and step or heel-toe back to Mountain pose.

VARIATIONS

- The arms don't have to spin 180 degrees to be parallel to the feet, they can be perpendicular, out in a T-shape. That requires less twist.
- This can be done with or without props. The firm support of a kickboard is especially nice for this pose.

- Check to make sure students turn their back toes in enough.
- Students often round their spine and then try and twist. They need to hinge the hips first, keep the back straight, and then, if there's space, twist.
- Remind students to be kind to their back shoulder so they don't strain it trying to raise their back arm.

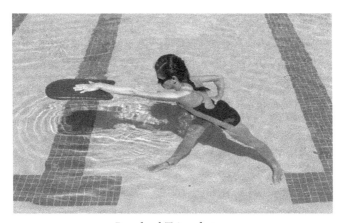

Revolved Triangle pose

Warrior I or Virabhadrasana I

For Warrior I pose, or Virabhadrasana I, start in Mountain pose. Step forward with your right foot two large or three small steps. Your left toes will still be on the pool floor, but your left heel will be raised. Both feet are still hip-bone distance apart, like on narrow railroad tracks. All ten toes are going the same direction. Inhale, as you exhale bend your right knee in line with your right toes. Extra weight on the outside edge of your right foot can help keep the knee from diving in. You sink straight down with your torso as you bend your knee, so your shoulders stay on top of your hips. Your arms go anywhere depending on the variation you're practicing. To come out, straighten the knee, and step back with your right foot into Mountain pose.

VARIATIONS

There are many choices with your arms based on what you want to emphasize. The arms can hold still or move dynamically such as:

- Both arms overhead (sagittal or coronal plane).
- Both arms on the surface of the water (transverse plane).
- Both arms down towards your hips or anywhere else through the water.
- Arms interlaced behind your back.
- Any asymmetrical combination of those to challenge your brain, in addition to your strength and balance.
- Do any of those arm combinations with props.
- Place a noodle under the front toes to learn to keep the weight in the back foot.

TEACHING TIPS

- I teach Warrior I with the back heel raised like Crescent Lunge pose (Anjaneyasana) because most of the students I teach don't have the flexibility in their hips, back, or legs to be successful and safe with the traditional back heel down. You can absolutely teach Warrior I the traditional way with the back heel down and the hips rotated, if that works for your people.
- Some students need to bend the back knee. That's fine. Still encourage reaching through the back heel to maintain their stability in the posture.

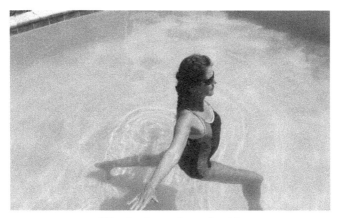

Warrior I pose from the side

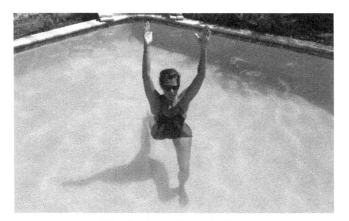

Warrior I pose from the front

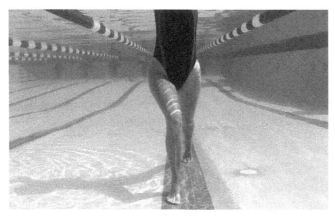

Warrior I pose underwater

Warrior II pose or Virabhadrasana II

There are two chief ways to get into, and out of, Warrior II pose or Virabhadrasana II, building on the ways you entered Triangle and Warrior I pose.

Starting variation one: Take a wide-legged stance with parallel feet. Turn the toes on the right foot out to be at a right angle to the left. Pivot the left toes a little closer towards the right toes. Proceed as below. To switch sides, bring the feet back to parallel in center, and pivot to the other direction. Pivot back to the center and come out through wide-legged Mountain pose.

Starting variation two: In Mountain pose, take one, two, three steps forward with your right foot. Pivot out slightly on the left toes to anchor your back heel. Proceed as below. Step back with your right foot to the center. Step forward with your left foot to do the other side and come out through Mountain pose.

In both variations, your arms open up to be approximately wrists above ankles. In variation two, this will require you to rotate your hips. Bend the knee on the right foot in line with the right toes. Weight on the outer edge of your right foot makes this easier. Your torso sinks straight down as you exhale. Keep your shoulders back over your hips. You can look over the right hand or in the same direction as your belly button. You straighten the knee and step the feet back together to end up in Mountain pose.

See Exalted Warrior/Humble Warrior pose for Warrior II variations.

TEACHING TIPS

- Use the cueing variation that creates the smoothest transition from your last, or into your next, pose.

- Encourage more weight on the outer edge of the bent knee foot so students keep their knee in line with their hips.
- Students always put too much weight in the front foot. Encourage as much as weight as possible on the back foot. Using a noodle under the front toes as in Warrior I can help teach this.

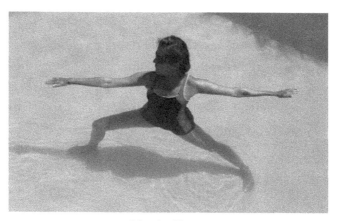

Warrior II pose

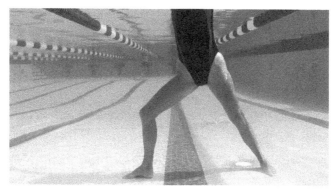

Warrior II pose showing good knee alignment underwater

Exalted Warrior/Humble Warrior pose or Viparita Virabhadrasana/Baddha Virabhadrasana

For Exalted Warrior pose, or Viparita Virabhadrasana:

From Warrior II pose, inhale and raise the right arm up overhead. Lower the left hand down to your straight leg. If you're doing this with a prop in the bottom hand, it's resisting buoyancy and strengthening the bottom arm. If you're doing this with a prop in the top arm, you're resisting gravity and strengthening the top arm.

For Humble Warrior pose, or Baddha Virabhadrasana:

From Warrior II pose, exhale and lower the right hand towards the knee. Raise the left hand up. If you're doing this with a prop in the bottom hand, it's resisting buoyancy and strengthening the bottom arm. If you're doing this with a prop in the top arm, you're resisting gravity and strengthening the top arm. In both variations, look where you want to look. To come out, follow the directions from Warrior II.

VARIATIONS

- These poses can be done with or without props in one or both hands.
- Putting a noodle under the front toes helps teach keeping the weight on the back foot.

TEACHING TIPS

- Cue alignment for the front hip, knee, and toes to all face the same direction.
- Humble Warrior with a buoyant prop in the lower hand is the hardest variation. Students struggle with getting the prop underwater and lose their form. Sliding the noodle down against the body is less effort than lowering the noodle with a straight arm.
- Protect students' shoulders by offering variations like hands to shoulders, top of the head, or only moving one arm.

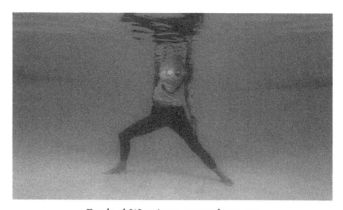

Exalted Warrior pose underwater

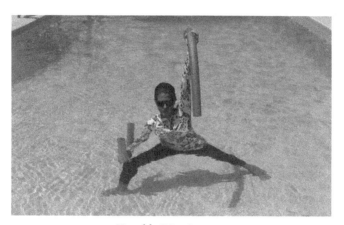

Humble Warrior pose

Goddess pose or Utkata Konasana

For Goddess pose, or Utkata Konasana, start in Mountain pose. Step your feet out wide, wider than shoulder-distance apart. Turn your toes out, at an approximately 45-degree angle. Bend your knees in line with your toes and sink into a squat. Look down; if your knees have come inside the plane of your big toes, either pivot on your heels to bring your toes closer together, or make your groin muscles work and bring your knees further out. Your arms can do any of the following variations. Straighten your legs and step your feet back together to come out.

VARIATIONS

There are lots of arm variations available in Goddess pose with or without props:

- Arms overhead in the sagittal or coronal planes.
- Transverse arm movements.
- Triceps and biceps curls.
- Circle a prop around you with a hand switch in front and/or behind.
- Bring straight arms together through the water in front or behind you, or, alternating one hand behind and one hand in front.
- Use Goddess pose to relax and release your hips by "hula hooping" your Goddess. Once you're in the pose, circle your hips in one direction and then the other.
- Shift the weight to one side, bending that knee more and straightening the other leg. Come through center and then go the other way.
- Bring Goddess pose to one or both tiptoes.

TEACHING TIPS

- Most students bring their knees inside the plane of their feet. This is hard on their knees and decreases their balance. Encourage placing the weight on the outside edge of the feet.
- Goddess pose functions well as a transition to floating meditation.
- For Ai Chi instructors, Goddess pose is the same base as you're using in your classes. Use these cueing techniques to get students to pay attention to their feet and have more ergonomic joint alignment in their movements.

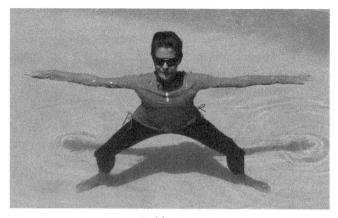

Goddess pose

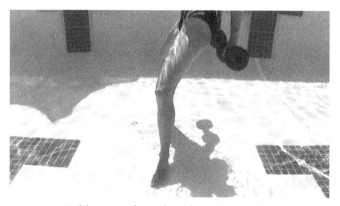

Goddess pose from the side with dumbbells

Gate pose or Parighasana

For Gate pose, or Parighasana, start in Chair pose with one noodle under each armpit and supporting your forearms in front. Or, if using dumbbells, your arms are spread out in a T-shape. Stay firm with your left foot and bring your right leg up. Cross it over the left so you're in cross-legged Chair pose. Lean your torso to the left as you come onto the outer edge of the left foot and straighten the left leg. The full sole of your right foot will come onto the pool floor and your legs are still crossed. If you look down at your legs, they make an X-shape. Inhale and pull yourself back up to your cross-legged Chair. Uncross your legs to come back into Chair pose and then straighten back up to Mountain pose.

VARIATIONS

- To turn this into a side-to-side flow, after doing Gate pose to the right, keep your right leg crossed on top in the center. Then, lean your torso to the right coming onto the inner edge of your left foot. Straighten both your legs to come into Side Plank pose with crossed ankles, outer edges of your feet together. Inhale, bend your knees as you pull yourself back up to center and cross-legged Chair pose.

TEACHING TIPS

- You'll need a chair or stool to demo this pose effectively on the pool deck.
- If people lose the cross of their ankles in Side Plank when doing the flow, that's okay but you'll need to remind them to add the cross back in as they come back up into Gate pose.

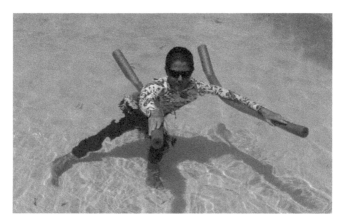

Gate pose

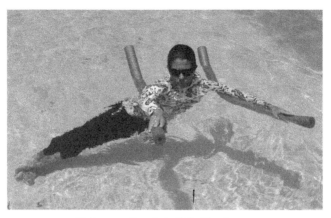

Gate pose flow into Side Plank pose

Sun Salutations or Surya Namaskar

Land yoga classes are often organized around what's called a flow. Flow in land yoga means movement with breath. For example, on an inhale you raise your arms up overhead into extended Mountain pose and then on an exhale fold all the way into a Forward Fold pose. The flow continues from there with each breath linked to a movement.

A flow in the water has to be inherently different because you move slower through the water. You can't complete the same range of motion, in the same half round of breath, in the water as on land. A flow in the water is more about moving literally with the flow of the water. You're timing your movements to your breath, but it might take anywhere from one to three breaths to accomplish one aspect of the Sun Salutation. As a teacher, it's important to try Sun Salutation variations before teaching them so you can feel the slower pace within your own body. When teaching, watch your students and cue at the pace they're physically able to move at. Don't get too far ahead of them. The following one-noodle Sun Salutation flow has the minimum full breaths (one inhale plus one exhale) in parentheses after the pose names as an example. Allow more breaths for beginners.

- Mountain (1)
- Extended Mountain (1)

- Cobra (2)
- Warrior II (2)
- Exalted Warrior/Humble Warrior (1/1)
- Cobra (2)
- Mountain (1)

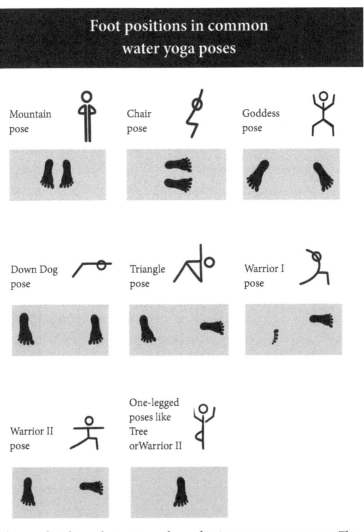

This graphic shows the position of your feet in common yoga poses. The orientation of the feet relative to the "yoga mat" and to each other stays the same in the pool, even though you won't have a mat for reference.

Balance poses

Four tips to better balance in water yoga:

1. When in Mountain pose, leaving your feet on the pool floor, lift all ten toes up. Note how your body comes back in space and your joints stack. Leave your body where it is and set your toes back down. In any balance posture, apply this toe lift to the standing leg, to help stabilize yourself.

2. In poses, your arms are usually floating on the surface. Instead of relaxed hands or sculling, bring the hands out into a T orientation (hands straight out of your shoulder sockets). Press down gently with your palms as if the water were a solid instead of a liquid. Notice how your torso muscles engage, and your stability increases. Remember this idea when determining which arm variation you want to do in a posture.

3. When performing balance postures, you put a lot of effort into the leg that is lifting. That adds to the destabilizing, rotational effects of buoyancy. For better balance, concentrate on keeping the opposite shoulder lifted. For example, when raising your right leg with your hands on the surface in a T position, work hard to keep the left shoulder parallel to the pool floor instead of dipping down. Also, engaging the left pinky fingers will help keep the left shoulder back. Controlling the shoulder and hands like this engages your torso muscles to reduce rotation.

4. Once you're established in your balance posture, apply a Root Lock (Mula Bandha), or a Kegel, while in your posture. To do Mula Bandha, think about the last time you were at a concert and had to use the porta-potty. If someone knocked on the door, you might have stopped peeing in a panicky moment because you couldn't remember if you locked the door. That action to restrict the flow of urine is activating a Root Lock. When you perform it during water yoga, notice how your concentration level increases and your pelvic region stabilizes.

You can use any, or all of these ideas, in any balance pose to help you.

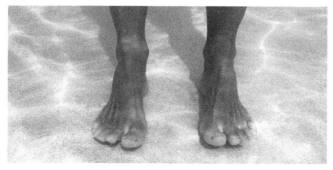

Lifting all ten toes up off the pool floor

Warrior III pose or Virabhadrasana III

For Warrior III pose, or Virabhadrasana III, start in Mountain pose with your arms straight out in front of you, thumbs rotated up towards the sky. Inhale in the center. Exhale and hinge forward in your hips while keeping your spine and arms long and straight. Your right heel comes up off the pool floor behind you. Keep the right toes pointing down to the pool floor. The right toes flex towards your nose as best as you can. Keep both hips parallel to the pool floor. Keep both legs as straight as you can. It doesn't matter how high the raised leg gets. You're trying to be one long line from your fingertips to your raised heel. Inhale while you drop your right leg back to the pool floor and straighten back up into Mountain pose to come out.

VARIATIONS

- Do this with or without any prop. One pool noodle under each armpit is especially supportive.
- Putting a noodle under the standing leg toes increases the challenge.
- Stepping back into Locust pose so the foot doesn't leave the pool floor at all is the most accessible version of this pose.

- Students tend to overrun their standing leg with their torso and hyperextend the standing leg knee. Ask them to pay attention to their standing leg. If their knee is complaining, suggest they shift their whole torso back a couple inches. That usually puts their torso back over their base of support.
- Encourage ankle dorsiflexion (toes to nose) on the raised leg for more stability in the water.
- Like in land yoga, students will raise the hip on the raised leg and turn those toes out. Encourage pointing the toes down to the pool floor on the raised leg. Also, the leg only raises as much as it can while keeping the hips parallel to the pool floor.
- Unlike on land, Warrior III with a prop in your hands is much easier in the water.

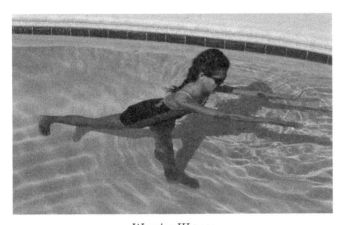

Warrior III pose

Front Leg Lift pose or Utthita Hasta Padangusthasana

For Front Leg Lift pose, or Utthita Hasta Padangusthasana, start in Mountain pose. Bend your right knee and bring the right toes to the pool floor. When you bend your right knee, your shoulders and hips stay parallel to the pool floor.

Option number one: Keep your right toes on the pool floor.

Option number two: Raise your right foot any amount off the pool floor with a bent knee. Your right toes flex back towards your nose, so your hip, knee, and ankle are all at right angles.

Option number three: After raising your right leg, straighten it out in front of you. Pull your right toes back towards your nose. Even if your leg is not straight, that's okay. Pulling your toes back towards your nose firms up your leg in the water and improves your balance. Your leg can be any height in the water, and it's okay to rest your right heel on the pool floor instead. When you're done, bend the right knee and set your foot back down in Mountain pose.

VARIATIONS

- The leg can raise into any position that works for you.
- Any props can be used in your hands while doing leg lifts.
- Leg lifts with either your back, or the sole of the raised foot, to the pool wall help teach alignment.
- Add a noodle under the raised leg, knee, or ankle. A noodle under the standing leg toes increases the challenge also.

TEACHING TIPS

- Students lean away from the raised leg to try and counterbalance themselves. Instead, encourage keeping the opposite shoulder lifted.
- Students tend to raise the lifted leg too high and shift their hips out of parallel to the pool floor. Encourage Ahimsa with good ergonomics.
- Some students lock/hyperextend the standing leg knee. Encourage a straight leg with a soft knee.

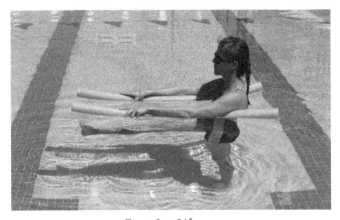

Front Leg Lift pose

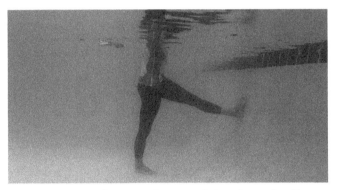

Front Leg Lift pose underwater facing the pool wall

Tree pose or Vrikshasana

For Tree pose, or Vrikshasana, start in Mountain pose. Be strong and stable on your left foot. Bend your right knee coming onto your right toes. Pivot on your right toes to open your right knee out to the side like opening a book. Connect your right heel with your left ankle. This is Tree pose option number one.

Option number two: Lift your right foot and connect the sole of your right foot to your inner left leg. The sole of your right foot can be any-where on your left leg except pushing against your left knee. Push your straight left leg into your right foot, as much as you push your right foot into your leg, so your left hip doesn't shift away. Only raise your leg the amount that works for you. Pick a focal point, a Drishti, in the distance to focus on. That improves your concentration and balance while in the posture. When you're done, straighten your right leg and pivot it back to the center to return to Mountain pose.

VARIATIONS

- Use a prop or the pool wall for support instead of freestanding.
- Use a noodle under the bent leg knee or the standing leg foot for a different challenge.
- While in Tree pose, sway your arms into a side stretch to make Palm Tree pose.
- For a flow, come into Tree pose and then step to the side into Warrior II pose. Bring yourself right back up to Tree pose. I call this planting acorns.

TEACHING TIPS

- Students tend to raise the foot of the bent knee too high and shift into the standing leg hip. Suggest keeping the hips parallel to the pool floor and maintaining equal pressure between the standing leg and foot.

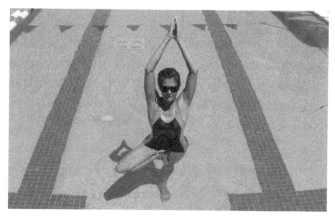

Tree pose

Side Leg Lift/Extended Hand to Big Toe pose or Eka Pada Padangusthasana

For Side Leg Lift/Extended Hand to Big Toe pose, or Eka Pada Padangusthasana, start in Mountain pose.

Option number one: Be strong and stable on your left foot. Bend your right knee coming onto your right toes. Pivot on your right toes to open your right knee out to the side like opening a book. Slide your right foot on the pool floor to open the right leg out to the side any amount. Straighten the right leg by pulling your right toes up to your nose while leaving your heel on the pool floor.

Option number two: After pivoting to open the knee out, bring your right knee up, so the thigh is parallel to the pool floor. Flex your toes back to your nose.

Option number three: After lifting your right leg to the side, straighten your right leg. Only raise the leg the amount that works for you. That can be returning your heel to the pool floor like option number one. Or for the greatest challenge, grab your right toes with your right hand. Anywhere in between is just as valid. Looking to the left adds more of a balance challenge. To come out, bend your right knee, swing it back to center, and set it back down to finish in Mountain pose.

VARIATIONS

- Do this with or without props in the hands.
- Doing Side Leg Lift pose with your back to the pool wall or the sole of the raised foot against the pool wall adds support and assists alignment.
- A noodle under the raised leg, knee, or ankle adds a new challenge.
- Flow between Side Leg Lift pose to Tree pose; or, flow from Warrior III pose to Front Leg Lift pose through to Side Leg Lift pose.

- This posture is more demanding of the hips than some. Make sure students are warmed up well for this.
- Remember, the leg doesn't have to leave the pool floor. The leg can be open out to the side with the heel on the pool floor.

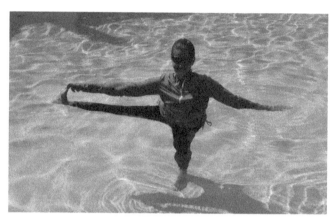

Side Leg Lift pose

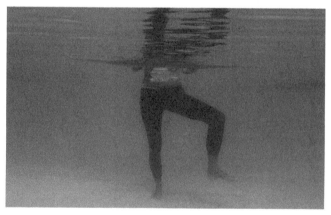

Side Leg Lift pose underwater

Half Moon pose or Ardha Chandrasana

For Half Moon pose, or Ardha Chandrasana, start in Triangle pose to the right. Shift your weight to the right foot and put a bend in your right knee. Raise your left leg off the pool floor, bringing the outside edge of your left foot towards the surface of the water as you straighten the right leg. Pull your left toes towards your nose, so your left leg stays firm in the water. Press down slightly with your right palm on the water's surface to stay stable in the water. Your left arm can be anywhere that's comfortable. To come down, bend your right knee and step well back with the left foot. Spend a breath in Triangle pose and then come up to Five-Pointed Star. Step your feet back together into Mountain pose.

VARIATIONS

- For more support, do this with props or with your back against the pool wall.
- Add movement with the top arm or leg for more challenge.
- Looking up at the top arm increases the challenge.

TEACHING TIPS

- When using a prop, students put all their weight into the prop and fall forward on the standing leg toes. Encourage keeping the standing leg hip above the standing leg foot to keep the joints stacked.
- Students tend to roll the top hip down towards the pool floor, then twist their spine to raise the top arm up. Focus on keeping the top hip back, and the top shoulder goes where it can. Encourage doing this posture with the whole back body stuck to a fridge like a refrigerator magnet.
- Students hyperextend the standing leg knee. Encourage keeping the knee soft or putting a teeny bend in it.

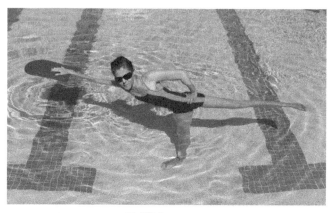

Half Moon pose

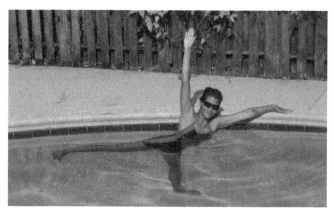

Half Moon pose with your back to the pool wall

Figure Four pose or Eka Pada Utkatasana

For Figure Four pose, or Eka Pada Utkatasana, come into Chair pose. Your arms are comfortably out to the sides in a T. Pivot on your right toes, and let your right knee drop out to the side. Cross your right ankle over your left. Your ankles are now crossed, and your right toes are on the pool floor. Another option is to bring the outside edge of your right foot onto the top of the left thigh. Anywhere between crossed ankles and right foot on the left thigh works. If you look down at yourself, you're the shape of an upside-down number four. To come out, return your right foot to the pool floor and straighten the legs to come back up to standing in Mountain pose.

VARIATIONS

- For more support, this can be done with your back against the pool wall or seated on the pool steps.
- For a balance challenge, Figure Four pose can be done seated on a kickboard or a noodle.
- The arms can be anywhere. Feel free to add variations and movement with the arms.
- Add one noodle under each armpit to make a suspended version of Figure Four pose.

TEACHING TIPS

- Joint replacements in the knees and hips are common so emphasize customizing this in a way that works for your students.
- To reduce strain on the ankle of the top leg, pull those toes towards that knee. The ankle dorsiflexion stiffens the joint and reduces lateral strain.

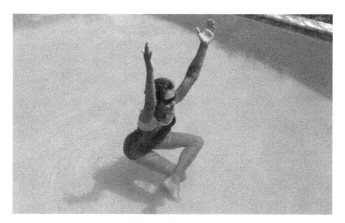

Figure Four pose

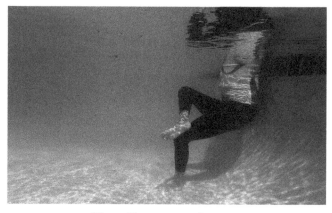

Figure Four pose underwater

Eagle/Cow Face pose or Garudasana/Gomukhasana

The names for these postures come from the action of the arms. You actually have three options for the legs in the pool. Combine the arm and leg positions in ways that make sense for your class and students.

Leg option number one: Chair pose.

Leg option number two: Figure Four pose.

Leg option number three: Traditional Eagle pose legs. Sink into Chair pose. Lift your right knee up to cross the legs at the knee, right over left. The right toes can support you on the pool floor, or you can wrap your right toes around behind your left calf. To come up, unwrap the legs and straighten them into Mountain pose.

Eagle pose arms option number one: Start in Mountain pose with your arms straight out in front of you. Your thumbs are rotated up to the sky, palms facing. Bring your palms to touch. Bend your elbows and bring your thumbs back towards your nose. For more stretch, raise both your arms further away from the surface of the water and bring your elbows closer together, or bring your thumbs closer to your nose.

Eagle pose arms option number two: Start in Mountain pose with your arms straight out in front of your thumbs to the sky. Cross your arms so your left elbow is stacked on top of your right. Bend your elbows, so both thumbs come back to your nose. Bring your right thumb closer to you so you can wrap your wrists, bringing your palms to touch. Again, arms further away from the water's surface, or thumbs closer to your nose is more challenging. Traditionally, the cross of the arms is opposite to that of the legs. These arm directions are for crossed legs with the right leg on top. Reverse the order of the limbs for the other side.

For adapted Cow Face pose or Gomukhasana, arms use one pool noodle. Hold the pool noodle in front of you with your hands wide towards the end of the noodle. Your thumbs are pointing towards each other. Leave your right hand where it is on the noodle horizontally in front of you. Rotate your left arm clockwise to hold the pool noodle from the bottom with your left hand. Both your thumbs will now point to the left and your left shoulder is rolled forward. Bring the pool noodle behind you vertically in the water by sweeping your right arm overhead and bringing your left hand behind your back. Both your thumbs will now be pointing down towards the pool floor. Draw your hands together on the noodle any amount you want. Unwind your arms to come out.

For Cow Face pose with a kickboard, hold the top of the kickboard in your right hand, looking at the back of your right palm. Swing the kickboard behind you, so your thumb is now near the back of your head and pointing to the right. You will need to apply some force to keep the kickboard against your back and not horizontal in the water. It helps to stand straight up and not round your spine or dip your head. Reach back with your left hand and grab the base of the kickboard with your left thumb against your back. Release the kickboard with the lower hand and unwind to come out.

You can also clasp your hands behind you without the noodle or the kickboard. Your legs can be in any of the variations above.

TEACHING TIPS

- Students find all this winding of the limbs challenging. Practice your cueing and break the movements down into small steps.

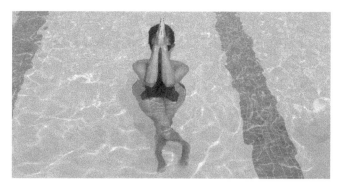

Eagle pose from the front

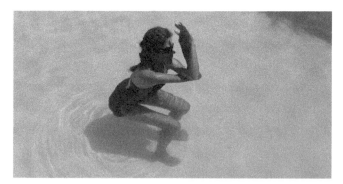

Eagle pose from the side

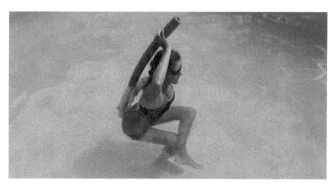

Cow Face pose with a pool noodle

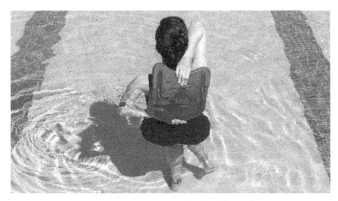

Cow Face pose with a kickboard

Dancer's pose or Natarajasana

For Dancer's pose, or Natarajasana, start in Mountain pose. Be firm on your right leg.

Option number one: Step back with your left foot and anchor the left toes like Locust pose.

Option number two: After stepping back, bend your left knee and raise your left heel back towards your bum, pointing your left knee down towards the pool floor, and your left toes up toward your bum. Your bent left knee is behind the plane of your straight right leg when seen from the side.

Option number three: After lifting the toes, your left arm reaches back on the water's surface, thumb towards the sky, as you raise the left foot toward your hand. Your hand may grab the inner edge of the foot, or not.

Option number four: After bringing the hand back, hinge forward in your right hip. Keep the knee of your right/standing leg relaxed and the foot grounded. To come down, release your left foot with your hand and place your foot on the pool floor. Use a focal point to increase your concentration.

VARIATIONS

- The standing leg arm can be in front, to the side, or raised up overhead.
- Hinge forward in the standing leg hip or stay standing straight up.
- Whether or not your hand and foot touch, actively engage the muscles that move your raised limbs together for more stability.

TEACHING TIPS

- While the traditional Dancer's pose is a challenging posture, there are many options to make this pose accessible to everyone. See more options for breaking down Dancer's pose in Chapter 10 when teaching mixed-level classes.

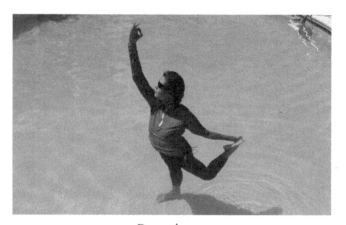

Dancer's pose

Prone and supine poses
Plank pose or Phalakasana

For Plank pose, or Phalakasana, with two hands on one prop (like one pool noodle) start in Mountain pose. Have your hands shoulder-distance apart on the noodle. Bring the noodle straight down in front of you, thumbs against your thighs. Step back with one foot, anchor your toes, and straighten that leg. Keeping both arms straight with the noodle weighted, step back with the other foot. You're now on all ten toes with straight legs. You're one long line from the crown of your head reaching back to your heels.

For Plank with two props, such as two pool noodles or dumbbells, start in Mountain pose. Bring the props down alongside your thighs, palms facing in. Step back the same as above, bringing your toes behind you. Keep the props under your shoulders with straight arms. When using the pool wall or steps for Plank pose, make sure your hands are shoulder-distance apart and step back with your feet.

VARIATIONS

- Take your Plank pose into a push-up by bending your elbows and bringing the prop in towards your chest, and then straightening your arms back into Plank pose. Keep your elbows tucked in towards your torso as you do this.
- With a prop in each hand, like when using dumbbells, take your Plank into lateral flies by opening your barbells up to the surface of the water, turning your body into a big letter T, and then bringing the barbells back beneath you to Plank pose.
- You can also roll this to the side for Side Plank pose and/or flow between Plank pose and Side Plank pose.

TEACHING TIPS

- If students bend their elbows or knees, it will roll their torso and they'll fall out of the pose. Encourage long and straight limbs, like a board.
- Sometimes students bring their props up towards the surface of the water. While that's a fine way to do Plank pose, it takes more torso engagement and control to prevent sagging in the

hips and low back pain. Encourage keeping the hands under the shoulders and perhaps offer a more buoyant prop instead.

- When people struggle with Plank on land, they let their hips sag. In the pool, they do the opposite. They keep their hips in flexion, with bent knees and with their bum closer to the surface of the water. Encourage trusting the props, engaging the gluteus muscles, and reaching through the heels to ground their feet.

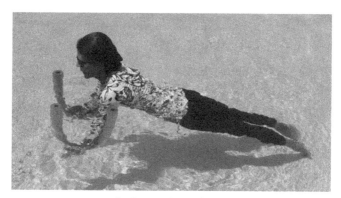

Plank pose from the side

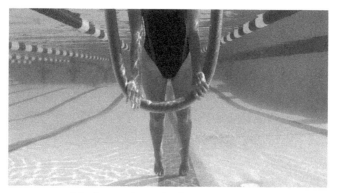

Plank pose from the front underwater

Cobra/Up Dog pose or Bhujangasana/ Urdhva Mukha Svanasana

For Cobra pose, or Bhujangasana, start in Plank pose. Once you're stable in Plank pose, one at a time, shift your feet so you're on the tops of your feet instead of the tiptoes. This will grind off your pedicure.

For Up Dog pose or Urdhva Mukha Svanasana, come into Cobra pose. Exhale and draw your hips towards the wall or pool floor to lift your chest. This accentuates the back arch you started in Cobra pose. Up Dog is often easier with a prop in each hand.

Where you position a prop affects where you feel this in your back. Lower in the water, closer to your torso, requires more of your low back. Closer to the water's surface is more upper back. Self-select which is better for you. To come out, bend one knee and ground your foot again. Step forward with the other foot, coming back into Mountain pose.

VARIATIONS

- Do this with one or two props, or at the pool wall.
- The difference between Cobra and Up Dog poses in the water is where you're placing your upper body and how much your back is arching. In both poses, you're on the tops of your feet.

TEACHING TIPS

- People will bend their elbows or knees, which will roll their torso, and they'll fall out of the pose. Encourage keeping the hands under the shoulders with straight arms and straight legs.
- Bearing weight on the top of the feet will often cause foot cramps. It's okay to do this on the top of the foot with one foot, and on tiptoes with the other, in preparation for using the tops of the feet on both sides.
- The difference between Cobra and Up Dog is also dependent on the water depth. Deeper water will yield hardly any difference. In shallower water, the increased lift and arch of Up Dog pose is more apparent.

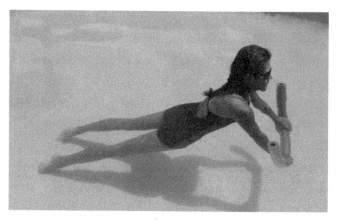

Cobra pose

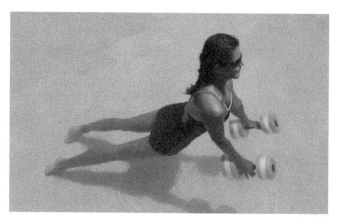

Up Dog pose

Child's pose or Balasana

For Child's pose, or Balasana, use two pool noodles. Thread one pool noodle behind your knees. Bend your knees and draw them up so you're floating in the water. Your other noodle is in front of you, under your wrists or in your hands. Lengthen your spine by reaching your fingertips away from your bum. Your feet stay under your bum. You'll need to find just the right balance point while lengthening. Look down at the surface of the water and keep your neck relaxed.

VARIATIONS

- Twist your Child's pose by pretending there is a stripe on the pool floor under your feet. If you gently swing your feet from side to side along the pretend stripe underneath you, you will gently twist your torso in the water.
- Get some diagonal stretch by reaching further away with the right fingers from the left buttock. Your right hip will drop in the water. Come back to the center and reverse to stretch the other diagonal.
- You can also do this at the pool wall holding on to the edge. One noodle still goes behind the knees.

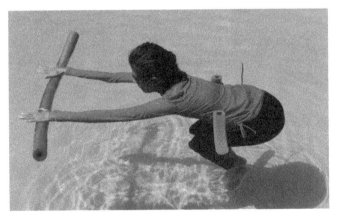

Child's pose

TEACHING TIPS

- People will be afraid of the water and stay very upright instead of flattening out to lengthen their spine. Encourage them to trust the props and find their point of balance, relaxing the neck and breathing through the nose.
- If people let their legs straighten, instead of keeping their knees drawn up, they will fall out of the posture. Go slow and encourage them to find their point of balance in the water.

- Bent knees with feet under the head is the cue for keeping people stable.

Reclined Hero/Camel pose or Supta Virasana/Ustrasana

For Reclined Hero pose, or Supta Virasana, use two pool noodles, ideally one normal and one large. Two regular noodles can be used in place of one large one—it's just more noodles to manage. Thread the larger noodle behind your back, and put the smaller one under your armpits. Bend your knees to weight the noodles and then straighten out to float on your back. Use your hands to bring the large noodle down to be at the base of your floating ribs. Bend your knees back as you bring your arms under your torso towards your feet. You can choose to grasp both, one, or neither of your feet. Keep your neck relaxed. To come out of the pose, let go of your feet. Straighten your legs while you hinge forward in your hips to come back up to standing.

VARIATIONS

- Reclined Hero pose can also be practiced in the zero-entry area of the pool as a traditional variation of the posture.
- Add a third pool noodle behind the knees to give a little more space and comfort.
- Try a standing version of Reclined Hero by bringing your back to the pool wall and opening your arms onto the pool deck in a T. Bend your right knee back towards your bum. Point your right toes and bring your heel tight into your bum. Your right shin will be against the pool wall. You might need to hop back slightly with your left foot to anchor your right shin. Raise your arms overhead and possibly bring them back into a gentle back arch by reaching for your right toes. Repeat on the other side.
- For a standing Camel pose, bring your back to the pool wall. Put your arms back behind you, placing your hands on the pool lip, fingers facing down. Your elbows face up towards the sky, shoulder-distance apart. Lift your chest as you walk your feet

away from your hands, which controls the arch in your back. Keep your feet facing forward and hip bone distance apart as they move away from the pool wall. To come out, walk your feet back under you, release your hands from the pool deck, and come back up to standing.

TEACHING TIPS

- This pose is best for people who are comfortable in the water. It requires getting your hair wet and some ability to maneuver around on the noodles.
- It is also demanding of people's knees and back, so consider your audience.
- I only offer this pose when appropriate for private sessions and use it in my personal practice.

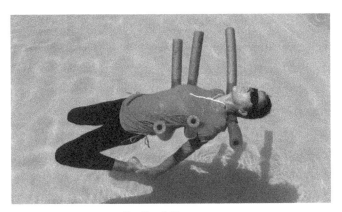

Reclined Hero pose

Seated poses

In land yoga, seated poses are thought of as grounding, restorative, passive, and potentially relaxing. In water yoga, you can use the zero-entry area to recreate the same poses and feelings, or move the seated poses into the center of the pool. In the center of the pool, almost everything about the pose will be different.

The zero-entry area of the pool, being shallow, recreates the feeling of seated poses on a mat with some water surrounding you. However, most of your classes will be too large to accommodate a group in that space. Also, people came to you for water yoga and probably don't want to get up and down off the pool floor. Save that section of the pool for your own practice or private sessions.

The most stable buoyant prop is to take one pool noodle and slide it between your legs to get comfortable with it. Sliding one noodle behind your knees to recreate a swing, offers a seat with a bit more challenge. Using a kickboard as a seat is the most challenging. Some people will need to keep one or both hands on the kickboard while using it. Use the prop arrangement that makes sense for your students with these poses. Also, the progression of these prop suggestions requires an increasing ability to sit upright. That requires engaging the core with enough length in your hamstrings to form an L-shape in the water; shoulders stacked on top of your hips.

Staff pose or Dandasana

For Staff pose, or Dandasana, take a seat on whichever prop you want to use. Bend your knees so you're suspended in the water. Keep your shoulders on top of your hips. Your arms can be out in a T-shape. Straighten your legs in front of you. Keep the inner edges of your feet together and your toes pulling back towards your nose. Strongly engaging your legs makes it easier to stay upright. To come down, bend your knees, ground your feet, and come back up to standing.

VARIATIONS

- Offer Staff pose as a progression rather than moving straight into the pose. Start with both knees bent. Straighten one leg at a time, alternating the legs. Then, bend and straighten both legs together. Finally, offer holding both legs straight out together.
- Offer any arm variation that works in your sequence.

TEACHING TIPS

- As you're learning seated postures, some sculling with the hands can really help. As students get more comfortable with all of these seated postures, they'll be able to do them with quieter hands.

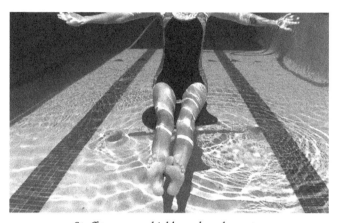

Staff pose on a kickboard underwater

Wide-Legged Seated Forward Bend or Upavista Konasana

For Wide-Legged Seated Forward Bend pose, or Upavista Konasana, start in Staff pose. Add opening the legs out wide and holding them there. Your shoulders stay on top of your hips, and your toes point up towards the sky while you simultaneously pull them back towards your nose.

VARIATIONS

- Make this a dynamic pose by scissoring the legs open and closed.
- Emphasize the action of closing the legs (to strengthen the adductors) instead of opening them.

TEACHING TIPS

- Start people off with the action in their legs before offering arm variations such as opening and closing the arms simultaneously with the legs.

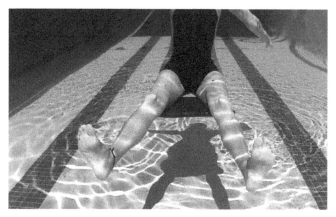

Wide-Legged Forward Fold pose on a kickboard

Lord of the Fishes or Matsyendrasana

For Lord of the Fishes pose, or Matsyendrasana, start in Staff pose. Bend your right knee into your chest more. You can stay here with the inner edge of your right foot glued to your straight leg or cross your right leg over the left to glue the outer edge of the right foot to the straight leg. Now your left leg, your hips, and shoulders are all pointing in the same direction. Add a twist by turning in your waist to bring the outside edge of your left arm to somewhere on the outside of your right leg. Your right arm can be anywhere. On the surface of the water in a half T-shape is the most supportive place.

TEACHING TIPS

- Twisting while floating in the water is challenging because there is no fixed point to twist against. Your body tends to roll in the water. Students need to have a lot of body control to do this posture because they have to recreate a fixed point within themselves.

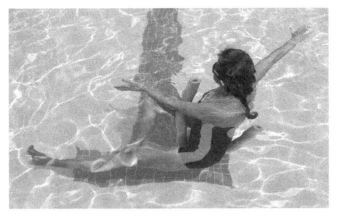

Lord of the Fishes pose on a pool noodle

Butterfly or Baddha Konasana

For Butterfly pose, or Baddha Konasana, take a seat on whichever prop you want to use. Bend your knees so you're suspended in the water. Your arms are out in a T-shape. Open your knees out to the side like opening a book and bring the soles of your feet together. Keep your shoulders on top of your hips and try to get the inner edges of your feet parallel to the water's surface. Drawing your heels towards your groin while pressing the soles of your feet together helps.

VARIATIONS

- Put one noodle under each armpit instead to do this posture in a vertical orientation. Leave the legs long, open the knees out to the sides, and bring the soles of the feet together. Point the toes towards the pool floor if you're suspended, or rest them on the pool floor for a more grounded feeling.

TEACHING TIPS

- Because there is less gravity pulling the legs apart in the water than on land, students tend to bring the inner edges of their feet together and not open their legs very much. Encourage pressing the soles of the feet together to add stability and a stretch for the groin.

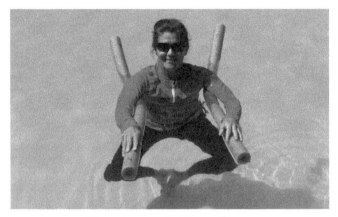

Vertical suspended Butterfly pose

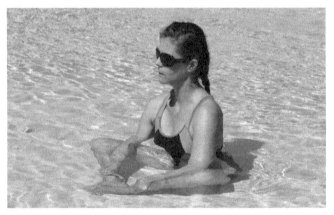

Seated Butterfly pose in the zero-entry area

Poses at the wall

Half Child's/Standing Pigeon pose or Balasana/Kapotasana

For Half Child's/Standing Pigeon pose, or Balasana/Kapotasana, start in Mountain pose facing the pool wall with your hands on the pool deck.

Half Child's pose option number one: Inhale and bend your right knee. Bring it towards the surface of the water, pulling your toes back towards your nose so your hip, knee, and ankle are flexed. Place the tips of your right toes against the pool wall.

Half Child's pose option number two: Instead of placing the tips of your right toes against the pool wall, point your toes and bring the top of your right foot and the front of your shin against the pool wall. You will probably have to bring your standing leg closer to the pool wall to keep it directly under you.

Standing Pigeon pose: Come into Half Child's pose option number two. Instead of leaving your right shin against the pool wall, cross your right leg over the midline of your body to the left. Some part on the outside edge of your right knee or your right calf will now be against the pool wall.

In all versions, your torso can remain upright, or you can drape your torso over the pool deck. Pad your forehead with your hands. To come out, lift your head up and lower your leg back to the pool floor.

VARIATIONS

- Shift your hands along the pool wall in either direction to turn this into a twist.
- Make this a flow by coming into Half Child's pose and then extending the leg back into Locust and looking up towards the sky.

TEACHING TIPS

- Students can splash some water out of the pool onto the pool deck if it's too hot for their arms.
- When doing the Standing Pigeon version, students sometimes report discomfort in the standing leg knee. That's usually due to torquing the knee when coming into the position. Encourage Ahimsa and never forcing positions.

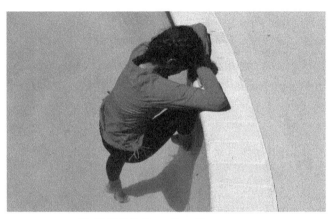

Half Child's/Standing Pigeon pose

Baby Bug pose or Ananda Balasana

For Baby Bug pose, or Ananda Balasana, start in Mountain pose facing the pool wall with your hands on the pool deck. Bend your right knee and shift the leg out, so your right knee is outside your right elbow. Bend your right knee more and bring any amount of the sole of your right foot onto the pool wall. Your toes will probably be turned out. That's okay. Bend your left knee and bring it outside your left elbow. Place any amount of the sole of your left foot onto the pool wall. Your feet are much wider than your hands. Both your knees are bent. Your fingers will be supporting your weight through friction on the pool deck, squeezing the pool lip, or hanging onto the pool rail if your pool has one around the edge. To come down, lower one leg back to the pool floor and then the other.

VARIATIONS

- Do this one leg at a time, alternating the legs, so both feet don't leave the pool floor.
- If you're hanging on the pool deck, alternate straightening one leg and bending your other knee more to take this side to side.

TEACHING TIPS

- This pose is actually easier with wide legs than legs together. Tell students that and encourage wide legs with bent knees.
- Some people find the idea of hanging from the pool deck scary. Acknowledge it's scary and reassure them that it's easier than it looks or sounds.
- Also, this position is unusual. People don't always act on your directions. If I'm on the pool deck, I'll do Baby Bug on my back to help show what's going on. If I'm in the pool, I do it with people.
- Once people are in the pose, they really like it. Try to juggle the cautiousness and enjoyment, and don't rush this pose.

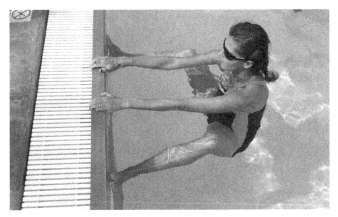

Baby Bug pose

Forward Fold pose or Uttanasana, and Wide-Legged Forward Fold pose or Prasarita Padottanasana

There are several variations of Forward Fold pose, or Uttanasana, and Wide-Legged Forward Fold pose, or Prasarita Padottanasana, you can practice.

Supported against the pool wall: Bring your back comfortably to the pool wall and support your torso with your arms in a T. Step one leg in front of you, straighten it, and press the sole of your foot into the pool floor. Straighten the other leg with the first. Alternatively, straighten your leg out to the side at a 45-degree angle, and then open the other leg to the other side for a Wide-Legged Forward Fold at the pool wall. Either of these versions can be done rocked back on your heels, and pulling your toes towards your nose. Your spine should be neutral. Don't overarch your low back or flatten your spine into the wall.

Seated on the pool steps: If your pool has steps, you can take advantage of them by recreating this pose in the same land-based form, with the benefit of having your hips submerged.

Freestanding: Step your feet out wide into a wide-legged parallel-foot stance. Keeping your spine long, hinge forward in your hips as much as you like. Having a prop, such as a noodle in your hands, makes this easier. This is exactly the same as the Down Dog pose.

Suspended on the pool wall: Start by coming into Baby Bug pose. Then straighten your legs and shift them out wider than they were in Baby Bug. Bringing the legs together, with the inner edges of the legs touching, is more challenging.

TEACHING TIPS

- In all variations of this, students tend to round their spine down and collapse their chest. Emphasize the folding hip action and keeping the spine long.
- Pulling the toes back towards your nose encourages the length in the hamstrings this pose requires.

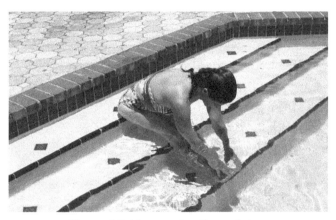

Forward Fold pose using the pool steps

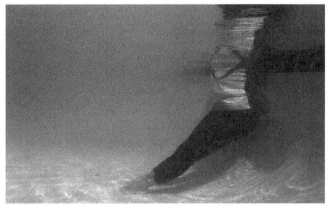

Forward Fold with your back to the pool wall

Side Plank pose or Vasisthasana

For Side Plank pose, or Vasisthasana, start in Plank pose facing the pool wall. Keeping your body straight in Plank, turn your whole body to the left like spinning a rotisserie. Come onto the outside edge of your right foot. Stack your left foot on top, bringing the inner edges of your feet together. Your right arm is straight from your shoulder to your base of support. Your left arm can be where you want. Keep your body perpendicular to the pool wall. To come out, roll forward back into Plank pose. Bend one knee. Ground that foot and come back up to standing.

VARIATIONS

- Place the top arm anywhere: straight up, straight out, or keep it parallel to your body.
- Raise the top leg up.
- Raise both the top arm and top leg.
- Instead of moving the top limbs and holding them in position, add dynamic movement.
- Do this pose in the center of the pool with a buoyant prop.
- Roll between Plank, Side Plank, Plank, Reverse Plank, Side Plank to the other side, and back to Plank, or any other order, as a rolling flow.

TEACHING TIPS

- When using a buoyant prop, students don't trust themselves or the prop and keep their knees bent. This will cause them to fall out of the pose.
- Students sometimes keep their tiptoes attached to the pool floor in regular Plank and then twist their spine instead. They should roll onto the outside edge of their bottom foot.
- Look for bent elbows in the supporting arm that will cause people to roll out of the pose.
- Cue neutral wrist alignment. Breaking the lower wrist back can cause discomfort.
- Students tend to roll their top shoulder forward, which disrupts

their balance. To help to keep the body long, they need to keep the whole back body parallel to the pool wall with the lower hand on a buoyant prop.

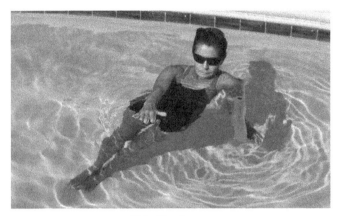

Side Plank pose

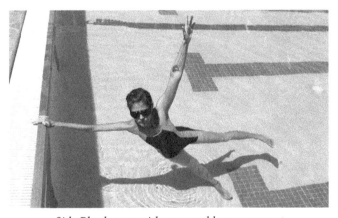

Side Plank pose with arm and leg movement

Reverse Table pose or Ardha Purvottanasana, and Reverse Plank pose or Ardha Phalakasana

For Reverse Table pose, or Ardha Purvottanasana, start seated on the pool steps. Place your hands behind you on the pool steps with your fingers pointing towards your bum. Bring the soles of your feet to another step or to the pool floor. Your feet and knees are hip-distance apart and facing forward. Lift your hips up any amount as you inhale.

As you lift your hips, don't let your knees bend past a 90-degree angle. Keep your feet pressed against the pool floor and roll your thighs in. Look straight ahead or up at the sky. Lower your torso back to the pool steps when you're ready to come out of the pose.

For Reverse Plank, come into Reverse Table. Straighten one leg out, bringing the sole of your foot to a pool step or the pool floor. Straighten the other leg out next to the first. Bend the knees one at a time and sit back down on the pool steps to come out of the pose.

VARIATIONS

- For a greater challenge, do this in the center of the pool with one noodle behind you perpendicular to your body, a kickboard, two pool noodles parallel side to side, or dumbbells.

TEACHING TIPS

- Most pools won't have enough room for you to offer this pool step version regularly. The prop variation can work for larger group classes.
- This pose is very challenging for most people's shoulders, forearms, and wrists. To make it easier, the fingers can turn out, the elbows can bend, and the lift in the hips can be minor.
- Students tend to splay their feet and knees out, which may aggravate an already sore low back. Encourage Mountain pose stance with feet hip-distance and parallel feet. The thighs roll in, and the heels push out.

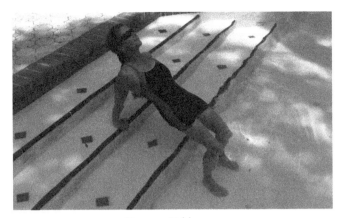

Reverse Table pose

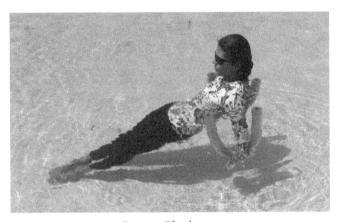

Reverse Plank pose

Chapter 5

Teaching Pranayama or Breath Practices

My partner is a marine ecologist, and he does damage assessments for oil spills. In his field, they have a joke, "The solution to pollution is dilution." Obviously, oil spills are bad but when a contaminant interacts with a large body of water, its impact is diluted. You can use this concept in your water yoga breath practices. When stress is contaminating your life, your breath and the water can be powerful enough to dilute it. That's why breathwork is the fourth wave of water yoga.

Prana means energy or life force in Sanskrit. Pranayama is moving energy around your body by using your breath. In the yogic tradition, the energy you're moving around with your breath isn't just oxygen and carbon dioxide but the vital cosmic energy that is in all life. In water yoga, Prana represents all the energetic possibilities in your body, including using your breath to affect your physical, mental, and emotional states.

Polyvagal theory, developed by Stephen Porges, provides a framework for how your body's physical, mental, and emotional states react and respond to your environment. The theory explains how you can be relaxed and happy one minute, and then distressed with a racing heart rate the next. Perhaps the only thing that changed was a noise, or someone in the next pool lane said something. Your primitive reptilian brain (your brain stem that controls things like your heart rate) will perceive a threat (perceive, not necessarily receive) and prepare you to take action before your rational mammalian brain (your neocortex that's helping you read this chapter) has a chance to register that the splash was just someone dropping a kickboard in the water and there's no need to worry about it. That lightning-fast engagement of your sympathetic nervous system developed to keep you alive in the face of danger from a predator, but it also feeds chronic stress.

All the daily inputs you receive cause your nervous system to react in some way. Those inputs are going to encourage your nervous system to put you in one of three places. I call them the safe zone, the muster zone, and the danger zone. When you're in the safe zone, you're calm and can engage with others socially in a fun way. You're enjoying yourself, and this is where you'd like to spend most of your time. The muster zone is when something you've consciously registered or not is causing you some distress and your nervous system has deployed its resources to keep you alert and vigilant to move you into the danger zone at a moment's notice. The danger zone is where your sympathetic nervous system is working hard, and your body has been flooded with stress hormones to cause you to fight, flee, or freeze.

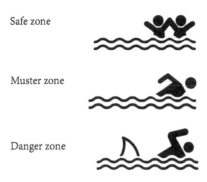

Polyvagal zones during water yoga

As a teacher, you want to make sure you keep your students in the safe zone. However, it's important to remember that the nature of the aquatic environment makes this even harder than on land. Students will bring the same daily stressors from life and mental health issues into their water yoga classes, but now they also have to navigate the aquatic environment. Despite the nervous system being dampened from the hydrostatic pressure, water yoga places a high demand on a student's sensory processing system. There's so much they have to pay attention to, both from a eustress (eustress is good stress like moving a muscle to build strength) and a stress perspective. Also, many people have a fear of the water. Just being in the pool puts them in the muster zone. You want to give people tools to manage their nervous system responses while they're in the pool, and in their daily lives. That's why Pranayama is powerful. Respiration is the only physiological response that is under your conscious control in any way.

Research has shown yogic breath practices can reduce stress hormones, anxiety, depression, and blood pressure. Pranayama can also improve your heart rate variability and stimulate the parasympathetic nervous system (the rest and digest system). All these effects help move your body from the muster zone back into the safe zone. Water yoga has the potential to create the same benefits.

To accomplish the physical act of breathing, your breath enters and exits your body through the effort of your diaphragm. Your diaphragm is a muscle that sits between your chest and your abdomen. When you inhale, it contracts, creating a vacuum that pulls air into your lungs. When you exhale, your diaphragm expands, and pushes the air out of your lungs. It functions like a pair of bellows, moving air in and out of your body.

If your lungs are fully submerged (a water depth covering your collarbones), it takes 60 percent more effort to breathe than it does on land. That's both because the increased blood volume in your thorax takes up space and the hydrostatic pressure requires your inspiratory muscles to work harder to expand your rib cage. Since breathing is more work in aqua yoga, there are teaching differences in which Pranayama practices we offer, how we offer them, and the impacts from these breath practices.

The following breath practices are easy for you to teach, and for your students to accomplish in the pool. No one breath practice is perfect for all people. Make sure your students know that if any of these practices cause them distress, they should return to their normal, natural breath. For students who live with asthma, chronic obstructive pulmonary disease (COPD), or another breathing condition, review Ahimsa. Encourage them to go slow, only do what's right for them, and perhaps work in a shallower section of the pool. These practices are listed in order of how hard they are to accomplish mentally and physically for your students.

Breath practices that are easy to do concurrently with Asanas

One of the simplest breath practices is breath witnessing. It's literally just noticing how you breathe. You don't try and change anything about your breath. Your normal, natural breath is keeping you alive and is perfect. You're just noticing when and how you breathe. For example, are your inhales and exhales the same length? Do you notice a sound when you breathe? Where do you feel your breath happen? As you watch your breath, does it change? It's getting curious about how you accomplish the act of breathing, and noticing everything you can about how you do it. Once you know how you breathe in the water, you can compare it to how you breathe on land. See if you can notice what the differences are for you.

Expanding on breath witnessing, you can label your breath. As you inhale, say inhale in your head. Say exhale in your head as you exhale.

Further expanding on breath witnessing, you can count the pace of your natural inhale and exhale. As you inhale, count the length of the inhale, and as you exhale, count the length of the exhale. There's no intent to change the rate. You're just counting the rhythm of your normal breath.

You can link your breath to movement. This can be done as a stand-alone practice or incorporated into any of your Asanas. Creating a relationship between your hands and your breath is an easy place to introduce this concept. With your hands on the surface of the water, every time you inhale, you rotate your palms to face up. Every time you exhale, you turn your palms to face down. The pace doesn't matter. It's entirely dictated by your breath.

You get to decide what that looks like for you in poses, but you're trying to be consistent. For example, when you raise your arms, you inhale. When you lower your arms, you exhale. You want to complete the movement at the pace of your breath. As you raise your arms, they would raise at the same pace as your inhale. Instead of sweeping your arms up fast and holding them there as you continue to breathe, the apex of your breath and movement happens at the same time. Another choice would be to step forward when you inhale and then step back when you exhale. The emphasis here is on consistency; consistency in repetition and timing.

Breath practices that are harder to do concurrently with Asanas

These are all options that involve altering the rate of your breath. It's easiest to change the pace after you establish what is normal within your own body. It's worth teaching the simple breath-counting practice first, before you offer these variations, so that your students have some familiarity with their normal breath and its pace.

Increased exhale: Make your exhale longer by adding a count of one as you exhale. The inhale is normal. Because a longer exhale stimulates the parasympathetic nervous system (the rest and digest state), this is considered a calming breath practice, and works well if taught towards the end of classes.

Increased inhale: This is a more challenging practice to perform than an increased exhale because of the hydrostatic pressure of the water. Make your inhale longer by adding a count of one as you inhale. The exhale is normal. Lengthening the inhale is considered a stimulating practice and it is therefore helpful to teach this when students are cold or have low energy.

Breath retentions: There are three options for breath retentions in water yoga. They're listed here in order of easiest to hardest to perform. Repeat each as many repetitions as are appropriate.

1. Hold your breath for a count of one after you exhale completely and before you inhale.
2. Hold your breath for a count of one after you inhale entirely and before you exhale. You will feel the pressure of the water more with this version.
3. Box breath – Inhale normally. Hold your breath for a count of one. Exhale normally. Hold your breath for a count of one.

While increased exhales, inhales, and breath retentions can be longer than one count, remember the increased power of Pranayama in the pool and add length only when appropriate.

Breath practices that work best as stand-alone practices

Sectional breathing (Vibhagiya Pranayama): On land, this is often taught as a visualization of segmenting your lungs into three sections. On an inhale, you fill the base of your lungs, then the middle of your lungs, then everything else. In the water, we have a distinct line dividing our bodies; everything below the surface and everything above. Because of the hydrostatic pressure, you feel the dividing line strongly. It's hard to inflate the lungs below the water, and as soon as you fill the lungs above the water, it gets a lot easier.

For water yoga sectional breathing, pretend your lungs are divided at the water level as you breathe. Inhale, trying to inflate the part of your lungs below the water. Feel the transition of underwater and above water. Inhale more, filling all the rest of your lungs above water. Exhale in the reverse order by emptying the part of your lungs above the water first. Feel the transition point the water creates. Expel the air out of the rest of your lungs. As you perform this breath, it helps to envision your ribs and breath spreading to the sides as you inhale. If feeling the spreading action is hard for you, place your hands on the sides of your body and as you inhale, try to expand your ribs into your hands. As you exhale, feel your ribs move away from your hands.

Alternate nostril breathing (Nadi Shodhana): I like to use a hands-free version of alternate nostril breathing in the pool because your hands are often filled with props, or moving through the water as part of your practice.

Start by trying to breathe through one nostril at a time. Begin by inhaling and exhaling through just your left nostril. Yes, some air will still come through the right nostril. That's okay. You're just concentrating on making it happen as much as you can on the left side. Use just your left nostril until you feel as if you can accomplish it. Once you're comfortable with the left, switch to the right. To the best of your ability, inhale and exhale exclusively with the right nostril. One side will probably seem easier, and that's okay.

Once you feel that you can isolate the right, begin to alternate the nostrils. Starting on the left side, inhale through the left nostril. Pause slightly at the top of the inhale. Exhale through the left nostril. Pause slightly at the bottom of the exhale. Inhale through the right nostril. Pause slightly at the top of the inhale. Exhale through the right nostril. Pause slightly at the bottom of the exhale. That is one round. Start again on the left side for the next round. It usually takes around five rounds to feel a little more comfortable with the practice, so allow enough time for your students to experience this.

Not all land-based yoga breath practices are good to do in the water. For example, Breath of Fire, or Kapalbhati breath, is a breath practice where you use your abdominal muscles to aggressively expel your breath. Some schools of yoga add in swinging your arms up vigorously overhead when you inhale and then dropping them back down as you exhale. However, the arm pumping breaks the surface tension of the water repeatedly and is not in alignment with best practices in aquatics.

Also, if your arm pumping action takes place only underwater, this becomes a balance practice instead of a breath practice. People with uncontrolled high blood pressure (their blood pressure is not under control through medication) shouldn't hold their breath in the pool.

Like all other aspects of teaching water yoga, it's essential to apply these Pranayama practices in your own practice first to observe their impact on you. Once you feel comfortable practicing each one, introduce it into your classes. Interact with your students to get feedback about which practices work best for them. As your students advance, continue to offer adaptations to the Pranayama options. That way, your students will understand how to customize the techniques for themselves and how to apply them to improve their practice, and life, in and out of the pool.

— Chapter 6 —

Teaching Pratyahara or Withdrawing the Senses

If the water meets the sea in an abrupt break, it's a cliff. If you try and get in the ocean from the cliff, it's stressful and potentially dangerous. You're better served by accessing the water from somewhere with gentler topography. Pratyahara serves as a similar gentler transition. As the fifth wave of water yoga, it serves us best when it's just a ripple at the shoreline.

Pratyahara is a concept that helps students shift between their external practice of the poses, thoughts about yoga philosophy, breathwork, all the hustle and bustle parts of the practice, and the peace of just existing in meditation like a flat turquoise sea on a sunny day.

As such, Pratyahara is a transition. It's an experience of exploring liminal space. Liminal space is a portal, an in-between place. Liminal literally means threshold in Latin. It's like the narrow strip of sand on the beach that gets wet from each wave coming in, the surf line. Below the surf line is the sand that is always underwater, and above it, the sand that is always dry. The surf line is always there; it just shifts in response to the context, like tides and storms.

Liminal or transition spaces exist because transitions are hard. Change is difficult. Pratyahara is about turning inwards to prepare yourself for concentration and meditation. You're withdrawing your senses from being focused on everyone else and what's going on around you, and tuning into yourself. Instead of stop, drop and meditate, it's gentler.

Pratyahara practices make some people uncomfortable, especially those who are more comfortable with the physical aspects of yoga. They ask students to transition from being outwardly focused on their poses and you as a teacher, to focusing on themselves and what's going on inside them. Your role as a teacher when teaching Pratyahara practices is almost like being an usher at the theater. When you enter a dark theater from the lobby, an usher is there to escort you to your seat and orient you to the space. The usher is a guide to help you navigate the transition from the lobby, where you had brightly lit cocktails and conversation, to the dimly lit magical story realm of the stage. Teaching Pratyahara helps people transition smoothly from the showy physical aspects of the practice to the slower mental aspects, like meditation. Have grace and patience with students who need to go slowly. This is an explanation I give to students who are struggling.

> We're used to relying on our senses. They keep us alive, and we need them. But they also bombard us and cause us stress. Practicing Pratyahara is not about turning your senses off; it's about slowing them down. You're learning to be less reactionary to your senses. You can't control your nervous system inputs; you can only control your responses to those inputs. If these practices are hard for you, notice that and try to practice them for one moment. That's it. Next time, try for two moments. Gradually increase the amount of time you disconnect from your senses so that transitioning into meditation is comfortable and natural. Just like the surf line at the beach is a flexible, responsive place, your Pratyahara practice is as well.

I think of Pratyahara as trying to find your personal channel on a radio. When you spin through the channels on a radio, some of the stations come in loud and clear, and some of them you have to strain to hear. You're learning to pass by the loud, blaring stations that are filled with advertising and listen for the calmer stations and perhaps even the deeper messages that come from inside yourself. As a teacher, you will find that this radio analogy also holds true. When teaching poses, you might be the loud, high-energy rock and roll voice on the radio, but you're the very quiet, night-time classical station host by the time you get to meditation. Teaching Pratyahara practices gives you a chance to transition in your teaching approach as well.

Practicing Pratyahara requires you to connect to more than your basic senses: sight, touch, smell, and so on. You use two big parts of your nervous system when practicing Pratyahara. Exteroception is being aware of everything outside your body. That's the sensory input you get from your eyes or the sensations of the water against your skin and the temperature of the pool. A Pratyahara practice is trying to shift your awareness from external to internal. Interoception is the felt sense of what's going on inside your body. It's becoming aware of your heartbeat and digestion, for example, but also your internal sense of movement.

There are two main components of interoception: proprioception and kinesthesia. Proprioception is your perception or awareness of the position and movement of your body. It allows you to move parts of your body without looking at them because you can feel where your body is in space. Kinesthesia is about how your body feels as it moves through space, what emotions are playing out in your body, how you feel inside at this moment. It's the felt sense of movement that allows dancers to be so expressive.

To put these together, imagine you're standing in the pool with your arms at your sides. Pretend you raise your right arm straight out in front of you until you break through the surface of the water. Your exteroception skills felt the water move against your skin, sensed you breaking the water's surface tension, and the temperature differential when your arm encountered the air. Shifting to interoception, your proprioceptive skills allowed you to raise the arm without watching it and controlled how fast you moved your arm. Your kinesthesia skills sensed how much muscular effort it took for you to move your arm. It told you which muscles were firing for your arm to move and sensed any physical discomfort, if there was any. This is a tremendous amount of information that your nervous system processes. How your brain interprets the information is where you can apply your yoga skills.

The fifth wave of water yoga asks people to shift their focus through all these inputs. Your students use exteroception, especially when they first get into the pool and feel the water. They use their eyes for the whole class to navigate the space. They use their interoception to move their limbs through the water to complete the poses through proprioception. Pratyahara asks your students to dig deep down into kinesthesia to be fully aware of how they're physically feeling. That sets them up to be comfortable within themselves to respond appropriately to the mental and emotional aspects of concentration and meditation.

Examples of Pratyahara practices to teach in the pool:

- Closing your eyes.
- Relaxing your jaw and letting your tongue rest gently behind your teeth.
- Letting your breath slow down.
- Experiencing the hydrostatic pressure of the water against your skin.
- Suspending drinking fluids.
- Practicing without speaking, instead of talking to a buddy nearby.
- Increasing the time you spend in postures and transitions to slow your practice down.
- Focusing on the internal aspects of your practice—such as the feelings of your internal organs, or the emotional responses you experience instead of the shapes your body makes.
- Exploring Svadhyaya, or the Niyama of self-knowledge as a Pratyahara practice.

One of the chief ways to practice Pratyahara on land is to close your eyes. But in water yoga, withdrawing your senses isn't just closing your eyes. Because of the increased safety requirements and the discomfort some people feel around water, closing your eyes isn't always an option. Fortunately, your nervous system is dampened down whether you close your eyes or not, because of the properties of water. The principle of hydrostatic pressure dampens the sensory input you receive from your nerve endings.

People who choose not to close their eyes are still practicing Pratyahara just by being in the water. This passive Pratyahara practice is enhanced even more by being in the deep end, since people will be more submerged. If people are comfortable in the deep end with their eyes open, you might encourage moving into that section of the pool in preparation for meditation. They will need a buoyancy aid in the deep end to maintain a passive, neutral body position. That can be accomplished with one or two noodles under each armpit or an aquatic flotation belt. If the noodles cause tension in the neck or shoulders, the flotation belt is a better choice. All flotation belts need to fit correctly—sitting low on the hips and tight. The belt should fit so that people can achieve a passive vertical orientation with straight legs and hip extension. The belt should never ride up so that it forces your students to roll their spines forward into a turtle shape.

A Pratyahara practice is hard to accomplish if people are cold. When people tune into themselves and the first thing they register is being cold, they're going to get stuck there at the first step of exteroception. As teachers, we can't control the pool's temperature, but we can make suggestions for swim clothes. Sun shirts, sun pants, and hats which reduce ultra violet exposure also help to keep people warm. Swim caps hold in the heat too. Thin neoprene shirts made for head-out water exercise work even better. If you know the pool is cold, transition into Pratyahara and meditation with a more active, physical approach to the poses, so that people are warm as they settle down.

Pratyahara is also harder for our students when it's loud and bustling at the pool. Do what you can to create a calmer, more peaceful environment for your students. You can ask bystanders carrying on loud conversations to lower the volume for a few minutes. Perhaps work with the pool staff to turn off mushrooms/jets/slides for just a portion of the class. Playing soothing music for your students might help drown out the sounds you can't control.

While withdrawing your senses and increasing your internal

awareness might sound slight and not worth emphasizing, don't discount this part of the practice during classes. I've worked with working moms, caregivers of ailing spouses, and vets who all say their water yoga practice is the only time in their day they get to focus on themselves. It's an opportunity for students to validate their internal reality. That's powerful, and one step in increasing their personal agency over their practice and in their lives.

As a whole-person practice, the skills you learn with each wave of water yoga build on the previous ones to create a suite of benefits. Pratyahara adds to the self-regulation skills students begin to form with Pranayama. Dharana, or concentration, the next wave of water yoga, takes people even more inward in their experience in preparation for meditation.

— Chapter 7 —

Teaching Dharana or Concentration

The definition of a wave is a disturbance moving through a medium. A wave can be energy moving through the air, or across the surface of the water. Stress isn't really any different. Stress is a disturbance moving through you. Some of those stressors are good and help you get things done. That's called eustress. Bad stress, especially when persistent, is harmful, and that's more challenging for all of us.

By increasing your ability to concentrate, you can choose which disturbances you want to pay attention to, and how you respond to them. Practicing Dharana, the sixth wave of water yoga, can help you become a good surfer of the waves of stress. Teaching deep concentration during eustress helps students improve all aspects of their water yoga practice. You can also help them use concentration to turn challenging stressors into perfectly tubular waves that give them thrilling rides instead of every stressor being a wave that crashes them down into a reef.

Have you ever held a seashell up to your ear to listen for the sea inside? Did you notice that all your concentration and awareness were focused on the shell when you did that? Even if you were on a busy public beach, the entire world was distilled down into that seashell for a moment. The distractions were all still there, but you chose to be completely connected to the seashell. Your curiosity and your focus were captured. You can use that same principle when you teach concentration during water yoga. You're trying to teach people to distill their focus into one area so completely that it doesn't matter what else is going on. People tend to think of concentration as a singular focus on one thing, in a pristine environment, and that distractions disrupt that focus. Because of that, deep concentration can be even more problematic for students in a busy public pool than in a quiet yoga studio. Part of your job is to help them see that distractions are always there and to give them a suite of tools to stay focused no matter what else is going on. The Dharana tools you can offer your students are mudras, intentions, positive affirmations, and mantras.

To make it practical for your students, Dharana is about deepening your concentration. Like most aspects of your life, everything in water yoga is easier when you concentrate on what you're doing. There are always distractions in your environment. It's your response to the distractions, and your own mental clutter, that are the barriers to your practice. These ideas are tools you can use to override those distractions or dive deeper into your practice. The techniques can be used to improve your balance and focus when doing postures. They can make your breathwork practice easier. A floating meditation is easier when you're focused, so concentration techniques can be used during your meditation or in preparation for meditation. Concentration techniques can also serve you in your daily life and be used outside your time in the pool.

Mudras are hand gestures traditionally used in yoga to direct energy within your body and help you concentrate. There are three mudras I teach my students to help them focus during class.

Not every aspect of land yoga translates exactly. Obviously, in land yoga, there is no mudra with your arms extended on the surface of the water. For simplicity, I've dubbed this Apas, or Water Mudra. When in Mountain pose, whenever your hands are on the surface of the water, instead of sculling, come into Apas Mudra. For Apas Mudra, bring the hands straight out of your shoulder sockets, as if you're making the shape of the letter T. Press down gently with the palms of your hands as if the water were a solid instead of a liquid. Use the slight lift in your chest to expand your breath. See if you can maintain the pressure with your palms. When your concentration wanders, you tend to relax your hands, wiggle your fingers, and collapse your chest down. Try not to let this happen as a solid body creates solid concentration.

Anjali Mudra is bringing your fingers and palms to touch, with your thumbs against your chest. If that bothers your wrists, bring the fingertips to touch with some space between the palms, and rest your thumbs on your heart. See if the pressure can be equalized across the whole surface area of the palm, fingers, and fingertips. By pushing your hands against each other, you'll be more firmly attached to the pool floor. The pressure of your hands against each other primes your feet to apply more pressure to the pool floor. Focusing on equalizing the pressure between your hands and your feet takes your concentration even deeper. Anjali Mudra can be taught in any Asana where the hands are free, or it's traditionally used as part of a salute at the end of class.

Chin Mudra is traditionally thought to evoke peace and concentration. It is done with the palms facing up and the index finger and thumb gently curled to touch. I like to offer Chin Mudra to my students during balance poses, which require a lot of concentration to physically hold the position. By offering a mudra also, it refines the focus away from the gross aspect of standing on one leg, to the more delicate awareness of one's fingers. It helps students to see that no matter what they're concentrating on, there are always opportunities to further refine their focus.

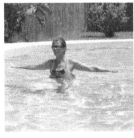 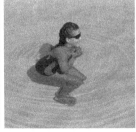 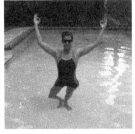

Apas, Anjali and Chin Mudras

The next three techniques are similar in that they all involve language, but they are each a different philosophical approach to increasing concentration. The traditional mantra is a word or short phrase you repeat over and over. It can be said internally, or verbalized as a chant. Like a mantra, a positive affirmation is a phrase you repeat over and over, but it is aspirational. A Sankalpa, or intention, is a personally created statement to keep your practice in line with your true purpose as an individual.

A Sankalpa is a practice goal that becomes a yardstick for measuring your level of concentration. Does each aspect of your practice align with your purpose in life? If your purpose in life is to live in empathy for yourself and others, a yoga philosophy intention would be, "Today I'm practicing Ahimsa and being kind to myself in all aspects of my practice." An Asana intention would be, "Today I'm working on keeping my head drawn back over my shoulders so my heart will stay open." It's easiest to introduce the concept of Sankalpa at the beginning of class and invite your students to create an intention for themselves. Once you're practicing, encourage your students to continue to check in with their intentions, both to keep their practice focused on their intention, and to maintain concentration. After class, encourage your students to note if their practice was in alignment with their intentions. If it got lost somewhere along the way, that's okay. It's an intention, not a law. That's why it's a practice, and why they want to come to class again.

Positive affirmations are a recent tool created by neuroscientists to help people change their behavior. A positive affirmation is a saying your students create to help them change something. It's the mantra equivalent of "Fake it till you make it." Positive affirmations work like the quote usually attributed to Henry Ford, "If you think you can, you can; if you think you can't, you can't." Your energy goes towards what you concentrate on.

For example, a common reason for coming to a water yoga class is that people want to improve their balance. They might say about themselves, "I'm such a klutz," "I can't even stand on my own two feet," or "Man, my balance is bad." What you concentrate on is more likely to happen because that's where your physical attention will go. Your concentration practice becomes your physical reality. If your students spend all their time thinking their balance is bad, how good can their balance get?

Your students can create positive affirmations to counteract negative self-talk, such as, "I am stable," "I am powerful," or "I am strong." Ideally, positive affirmations are short and sweet, so they're easy to remember and repeat. Obviously, they're focused on the positive. Like teaching Sankalpa, explain what a positive affirmation is and provide a moment for each student to set their own. Again, it helps to create the affirmation at the beginning of class to be a point of concentration they can use during the whole class. I find affirmations are often less personal than intentions, so there are effective opportunities to work them into partner work or even chanting.

The role of mantra chanting in group classes

Chanting is a very traditional Dharana practice. It allows you to focus all your concentration on one thing. It can be as simple as the traditional Mantra of Om, or one of the longer yoga chants. Chanting not only improves your concentration, it also has some other benefits. Chanting builds your breath capacity, almost like a hidden Pranayama practice. When chanting, you're not thinking about breathing as much as you're thinking about producing sound. However, projecting sound out, and extending the length of the sounds, helps you increase your breath capacity.

Chanting can increase your relaxation response. All vocalizations require an emphasis on the exhale. You don't make noise when you breathe in, only when you breathe out. Chanting increases the length of your exhale, which induces the relaxation response. Also, like any Dharana practice, it calms your thoughts, potentially reducing mental stress.

Chanting is also an opportunity for group work within a water yoga class. In a very traditional yoga class, the only chance for group work is a chant. Whether you run your classes as events for individuals or as highly interactive spaces, chanting provides an opportunity to connect with the whole group.

You can chant at the beginning of a class as a transition to a yoga space. You can chant between active postures and meditation. You can chant at the end of meditation as a way to mark the closure of the session. Where you place chanting in your sequence is up to you, based on your and your students' needs.

Here is an example of how I would lead a group Om chant:

We're going to chant Om three times as a group. You can join out loud and verbalize Om with us, or chant silently in your head. However you choose to chant, notice both the sound around you and how it feels in your body to vocalize Om. First, take a moment and get comfortable on your feet and in your space. Notice your breath. Smoothly inhale and exhale once in preparation. Inhale.

Om
Om
Om

Notice the residual effect of the sound vibrations and try to notice that moment when all the energy from chanting has dissipated.

What if chanting isn't going to work but you want the benefits of chanting?

Sometimes chanting is not an option. If you're coming to water yoga from aquatics, you might not be comfortable leading a chant. I haven't experienced it, but I've heard of facilities that won't allow chanting on religious grounds. You might feel your students aren't ready for chanting because of the associations they have with it. Here are three ways to get the benefits of chanting without the associations of "Omming" or using a yoga mantra.

A very simple chant that reinforces yoga philosophy can be done as a call and response. Tell your students you're going to ask, "Who's in charge of your practice today?" Ask them to respond with "I am." You can reinforce the call and response with hand gestures to help set the timing. Try for at least half a dozen times. This is especially effective when you encourage them to get a little louder each time. If you ask them to hold their hands over their heart while they do this, they can feel the sound resonance in their bodies in the same way they can with a traditional Om chant.

Song clip: If you include water yoga as part of a general aquatics class, you might be trying to sneak in some of the non-stretchy parts of yoga. For one of your song choices during the aerobics portion of the class, use a song that repeats one word frequently. Kool and The Gang's song, "Celebration," is an example. The word "C'mon" is used in that song a lot. When you're doing your aerobics, include having your students raise their arms and sing "C'mon" with the song as part of the chore-ography. Then when you transition to your yoga component and you want to add a moment of concentration, use "C'mon" again with the music off. Ask them to repeat "C'mon" loudly during an active stretch. As the stretches get slower, more passive, or smaller, each "C'mon" gets quieter. Eventually, they're saying "C'mon" only to themselves in their own head.

Verbalizing letters: Sometimes it's just the associations people have with the words Om or chanting that make people feel uncomfortable. Instead, you can ask people to verbalize letters. Explain you're going to work on building your breath by verbalizing letters. Start with A. Everyone makes the sound of A, several times loudly together. Then ask people to move on to U. U, in this case, makes the sound of yew, like the tree. After several repeats of U, move on to verbalizing M the same number of times. Once you're done, you can explain that these are the individual sounds of an Om chant. They had a chance to "chant" Om without actually chanting Om.

Dharana, or concentration, is the wave of water yoga that is easiest to apply outside the pool because it is universal and transportable. Helping students learn these techniques gives them valuable tools to improve their practice during class. More importantly, it teaches them how to apply their water yoga practice to all aspects of their lives, including for relieving stress, when they're outside the pool.

Dharana techniques can also be a meditation substitute for those people who aren't able or willing to do a full meditation practice, or experience adverse reactions during meditation. Research has shown many benefits of meditation for diverse populations. However, it's not a panacea. People with a trauma history, post-traumatic stress disorder, or mental health challenges are especially prone to unfavorable responses to meditation. Concentration techniques can be a bridge to meditation in a less triggering way—almost like "meditation lite." Usually, Dharana techniques are offered in addition to meditation. Still, for some people, they are a great replacement for a full meditation. Keep this in mind when you're choosing which meditation techniques you want to offer during your classes.

— Chapter 8 —

Guiding Floating Meditation

Floating meditation, or Dhyana, is the seventh wave of water yoga and is often people's favorite. It has the same goals as land-based yoga meditation described in the yoga sutras, to still the fluctuations of the consciousness. You're trying to guide people to achieve some peace and stillness in the midst of everyday life by learning how to do it in the pool first. There are some different practical and energetic considerations when meditating in the water, though. As a teacher, you need broad skills to lead meditations in the water because you have to introduce meditation as a concept, give directions for the mental aspects of meditation, and get people into and out of meditation positions safely.

Relentless—that's how waves are on the seashore, and that's how your thoughts are too. You can't stop your thoughts any more than you can hold back the waves. Meditation is not about stopping your thoughts. Meditation is about creating a little space between your thoughts, seeing if you can get them to slow down ever so slightly. You're trying to create the right conditions for that to happen for your students. Just as the waves are different on different beaches or with more or less wind, how can you create the right conditions for them to experience this?

When working with people who have no experience with meditation, I like to give them a visual explanation of what meditation is. I call it "Making it rain." While standing in the pool, bring your hands to the surface of the water with the palms facing down. Begin to splash the water with your hands. Your palms are churning up the water, and the surface is boiling now. That's what your brain (your hands) is doing to your consciousness (the water).

Begin to slow the action of your hands. Now your fingertips are moving on the water like playing a liquid piano. This is an example of how your thoughts begin to slow down because of your actions. Gently let your fingers still. Notice that the water is smooth and calm again. When your thoughts have slowed and calmed, your consciousness can also settle. Your brain is always bombarding you with thoughts. Meditation is allowing your raindrop thoughts to gently fall into the pool and dissolve into the fluid of your consciousness. You're moving from actively concentrating, to just being.

Offering floating meditations

There are three considerations when deciding which floating meditation positions to offer your students; prop availability, safety, and comfort.

You can only suggest what you have the gear for, so that's the first criteria.

If your students don't feel safe, they won't be able to get comfortable. You may or may not know if your students are non-swimmers, afraid of the water, or don't want to get their head wet. The vertical meditation positions are the safest because people's heads are out of the water. If people are uncomfortable in the water or getting their hair wet, start with one of those. If you do offer floating reclined positions, always include the directions for the upright positions first, for those who don't want to recline. Always give the directions for getting out of meditation positions, before the directions for how to get into them.

Lastly, we want our students to be comfortable to let their nervous systems relax. It helps to anticipate your students' needs based on your observations of their movement, what you know about water, and their body type. Some people might need the bigger diameter noodles when floating, for example. Remember to allow enough time with big group classes to help people get comfortable.

Part of being comfortable is also accommodating the conditions at the pool. People might need sunglasses to cut the glare, even with their eyes closed. A hat can shade their eyes and face. Suggest people grab their gear before they settle into meditation.

Not only do we need to support our students with trauma-informed practices, but we have the added element of water safety. Just like in land-based yoga, closing your eyes is always optional. If applicable, tell people the lifeguards are there and are always watching. Tell people you're right there on the pool deck, and your eyes are open the entire time. If needed, let people hold on to the pool deck, even if they're vertical with their eyes open, to help them stay comfortable.

Here is the order of operations for offering floating meditations:

1. Give directions for how to get out of the floating meditation position they'll be doing.
2. Explain what they'll be doing internally during the meditation.
3. Hand out props and let people get hats/sunglasses.
4. Let people know that closing the eyes is optional.
5. Encourage a calm, lowered gaze for those who leave their eyes open.
6. Give directions for how to get into their meditation positions.
7. Review keeping the feet under the head in vertical positions.
8. Help anyone struggling.
9. Play music if you're offering it.
10. Observe the students floating.
11. Give directions for how to come back up to standing.
12. Closing salutations.
13. Return props.

Explaining the mental aspects of meditation

Have a section of your teaching word and analogy bank that you can draw on when teaching meditation in the water. Just as you focused on strong action verbs when cueing poses, you need effective and evocative words when teaching meditation. Saying "relax" 12 times is not helpful. What can you say that is inspirational and concise to help people when meditating?

Examples for a meditative word bank:

- Contrasts: ebb and flow, rise and fall, rough and calm.
- Colors: from the black depths of the sea, to seafoam green surf, to turquoise lagoons.
- Other evocative words: salt air, sea breeze, swell, vast, iceberg, journey, voyage, trade winds, sunset, reflection, buoyancy, float, bob, diffuse, melt.

Find words that resonate with you and express the feelings, visualizations, or environments you're trying to create for your students. Insert these more expressive words for ones you repeat too often, or ones you've used that are more relevant to land-based work.

Creating analogies for the titles of your meditations can be a place to start. You don't always have to say, "Today, we're doing a breath-focused meditation." You could start by asking, "Can you grow gills in the pool today?" and follow up with concrete directions with the theme of breathing like marine life.

Here are some examples of meditation directions.

Setting your anchor deep

Anchoring within the various meditation traditions is connecting your awareness to a physical sensation. That helps you stay centered and focused during your practice. Today we're doing a vertical floating meditation. Once you get comfortable on your props, your toes might be against the pool floor the entire time or bobbing against it gently. If your thoughts or energy leave the pool and your practice, bring your awareness back to your feet and the sensations there. You're using your feet as your physical anchor to stay upright, your energetic anchor to stay grounded in your practice, and your mental anchor to stay focused in the moment.

The concept of anchoring while meditating is especially helpful for people who are afraid of the water. They can use their feet for safety and support. You can provide any physical sensation as a reference point for people to focus on. A Trataka, or candle-gazing, meditation can be beautiful to offer during outdoor evening classes as well.

Meditative scuba diving

An anchor point during your practice can be your breath. An advantage to using your breath as an anchor is that your breath is always there. Learning to use your breath to regulate your nervous system in the pool will help you learn how to do it when you're out of the pool. Because focusing on the exhale calms your nervous system faster, that's what you're going to anchor to. Combine a mantra with your breath practice. Every time you exhale, internally label it an "exhale." Let your body inhale and exhale naturally but when you exhale, you internally say "exhale." Inhale normally, exhale and repeat "exhale." Labeling your breath helps you stay attached to it as an anchor, so your mind doesn't wander down some other channel.

Any Pranayama practice can be offered during a floating meditation, so adjust your phrasing and directions to reflect what you're suggesting.

Don't get distracted by the baby shark song

It's noisy here at the pool. Instead of being distracted by the noise, you can use it as part of your meditation practice. Pick one noise to focus on. Maybe the flags in the breeze, the kersplash from the mushrooms, or the traffic on the bridge [insert the distracting noises your pool has]. All your attention is drawn to that noise. If the noise varies, take note but continue to stay attuned to the noise. If the noise comes and goes, use the pauses to focus on the lack of noise. Practice active listening while you're waiting for the noise to come back. This is not about getting sucked into someone else's conversation. You're not telling your own stories inside your head about the noise. You're simply witnessing the sound. Voices, splashes, tractors, airplanes, it's just sound. The power of learning to use noise as an ally is that it helps you when you're out and about in your daily life and are faced with loud distractions.

You can also play music and encourage people to use that as a point of focus during meditation. You can also encourage people to use an internal mantra or chant as their sound-based focal point.

If you want to offer longer, guided meditations, record them. You can play them using a sound system while people are meditating. That ensures that the volume will be loud enough for people to hear, and it will protect your voice.

Floating meditation positions

When cueing getting into floating meditations, work from the top down. Cue the props around the shoulders and head first, and behind the knees and feet second. That's because the lower props are destabilizing. As soon as people place those, they're floating. For safety, they need their head secure first.

When cueing getting out of floating meditations, start at the base and work up. First, remove noodles from behind the feet and knees to ground again. Then deal with the rest of the props. That gets people back on their feet quickly.

All vertical floating positions require the ability to keep your feet under your head. Non-swimmers don't recognize this and don't know how to roll their torso to return to a feet-under-head position if they get into trouble. Using a pool noodle amplifies this effect because of the buoyancy. If you let your feet come up to the water's surface in front of you, the back of your head will dip into the water. If you let your feet come up towards the surface of the water behind you, your face will get wet. Review this concept with your students when giving them directions. Tell them if either of those things happens, "Bend your knees, roll to the side, and bring your feet back under your torso." Emphasize the bending of the knees part of these directions.

The positions that follow are listed in order of how much gear they require and how easy and accessible they are. The upright positions are more accessible and need less equipment. The reclined positions are less accessible because they require more comfort in the water, more body control, and flexibility to manage the props. They also potentially need more gear. Because props facilitate buoyancy and relaxing, when you can, offer them. Since props are not always available, I give two solutions at the end of this list for prop-less meditations.

Using one pool noodle for support is the easiest option. One noodle can go against your chest in front and wrap under your armpits. Or it can be behind you, against your back, and under your armpits. Bend your knees to let the noodle support your weight. Some people will be fully floating here. Some will still have their toes attached to the pool floor. Some people will be bobbing and have their feet against the pool floor intermittently. All of those are fine, but remember to cue feet under the head for safety.

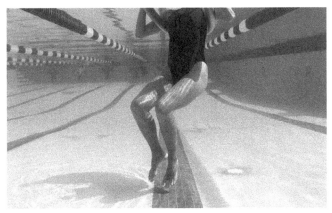

Floating meditation with one noodle behind your shoulders

You can also use two pool noodles in the same positions for more buoyancy, or for efficiency in managing props during a class. To come out, straighten your legs and come back up to standing.

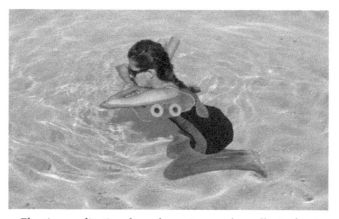

Floating meditation draped over two pool noodles in front

For more support but still keeping your head out of the water, you can ride a noodle bicycle. Take one noodle and thread it between your legs to get comfortable with it. Center yourself on the noodle. Settle your weight into the pool noodle under you by bending your knees as if you're sitting in a floating chair. Keep your feet under your head. Some people find that easier if they cross their ankles.

For more support, another noodle can go behind your back and under your armpits. To further support you, especially for tension in the neck and shoulders, the noodle can go under your wrists in front instead. These options can be combined as a three-noodle seated float to be even more supportive.

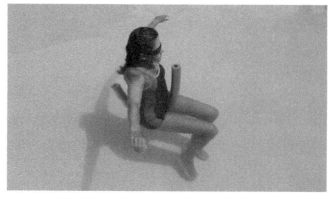

Floating meditation with a noodle bicycle

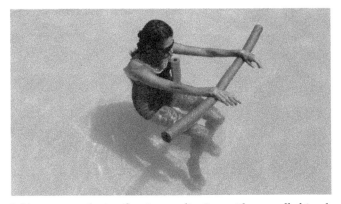

Wrist support during floating meditation with a noodle bicycle

Instead of a bicycle, you can thread a noodle behind your thighs like a swing. A second noodle behind you helps hold you upright. A third noodle can go in front here as well. This position requires you to pay more attention to your balance than the noodle bicycle version.

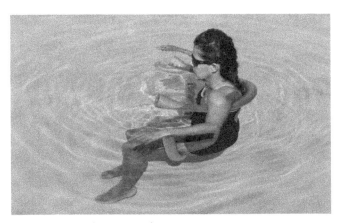

Floating meditation, as in a swing

If you used aquatic dumbbells during your practice, it might be most efficient to continue to use them during your floating meditation. You can place them under your armpits and bend your knees. You can also use the barbells under your armpits and add one noodle by getting comfortable with it, like sitting in a floating chair again.

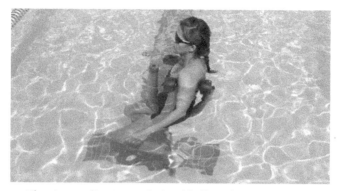

Floating meditation with dumbbells under your armpits

To come out of these seated positions, ground your feet by straightening your legs. Stand upright again and secure your props.

For students who struggle with back pain, there's a way to get some spinal traction and pain relief during meditation. This is best for people with some comfort with the water because they need to move to the deep end of the pool. Slide one or two noodles under each armpit so that the noodles are perpendicular to your body. Your forearms can rest on the pool noodles in front of you or on the surface of the water. Because your feet are off the pool floor, and the pool noodles' buoyancy is supporting your upper body, you're getting a bit of spinal elongation here. Visualize creating length and space during your meditation to enhance that feeling. To come out, swim back to the part of the pool where your feet touch, and remove the noodles.

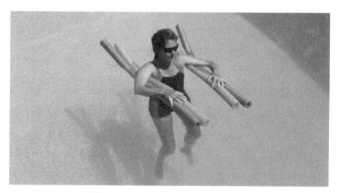

Vertical floating meditation for spinal traction

The reclined floating meditation positions are the most similar to a land-based Corpse pose. Start by threading one pool noodle behind your shoulders and under your armpits. Bend your knees and thread the other pool noodle behind them. You might be in a semi-floating chair now. Flatten out by straightening your waist and your legs. Your ears will probably be underwater.

If you want more support in a reclined float, use more pool noodles. When using three or four noodles, it's helpful to have them in at least two colors to make it easier to see if they twist around you.

For three noodles, thread two different colored noodles behind you and under your armpits. Bend your knees and thread the remaining pool noodle behind your knees. Once you've flattened out, use your hands to shift the higher noodle from your shoulders to under your neck.

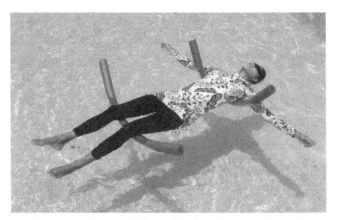

Floating meditation fully reclined with two pool noodles

With four noodles, start the same as the three-noodle float but thread two different colored noodles behind your knees. Once you're reclined, reach down with your hands, or use your feet, to move the lowest noodle from your knees to under your ankles. Use your hands to shift the highest noodle from behind your shoulders to under your neck. Your arms float comfortably on the surface of the water.

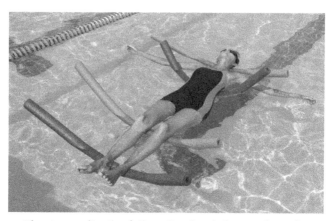

Floating meditation fully reclined with four pool noodles

To come out of all these reclined positions, remove the noodles starting at your feet. With four noodles, remove the pool noodle from behind your ankles first by shifting your feet off it. Then for positions with a noodle at the knees, bend at the waist and reach down to remove the pool noodle behind your knees. Come back up to standing by straightening your legs, and secure your props.

A very solid and stable position, but one that puts your head under the water, is to float with your legs on the pool wall. Stand near the wall with one noodle behind your shoulders and tucked under your armpits. Face the pool wall and hang onto the pool deck with one hand. Whichever side is hanging onto the pool deck, raise that leg and put your calf on top of the pool deck. Continue to hang onto the pool wall. Bring your other leg up, so both calves are resting on the pool deck. Let go of the pool wall. Your knees are bent, and your torso is on the surface of the water. The noodle can stay behind your shoulders, or you can use your hands to shift it to under your neck. Your arms go where they're comfortable. To come out of the position, bend at your side waist to bring one hand back to the pool wall. Swing your legs the other direction off the pool deck to ground your feet on the pool floor again.

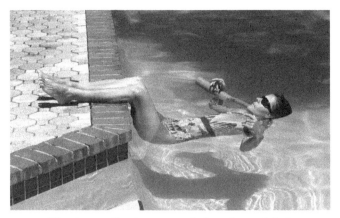

Floating meditation suspended on the pool deck

What if you don't have access to any props?

A standing, supported meditation is one option. Bring your back to the pool wall. Anchor your bum to the wall and walk your feet in towards the center of the pool. Your legs can be straight with the toes raised, resting on the heels, or with a comfortably bent knee and the soles of the feet on the pool floor. Slide down in the water, and more of your back will contact the pool wall. The arms should be where they're comfortable. Some people like opening their arms up into a T-position on the pool deck, so they help support a little bit of their weight. Some people like letting their arms float on the surface in front to emphasize the feeling of weightlessness. Another option is to embrace the torso in a gentle hug to increase the feelings of security. Close the eyes or leave them open and let the eyelids be heavy. While this is similar to a wall supported Forward Fold, you're trying to emphasize a passive, relaxing release here rather than an active posture with an aggressive stretch.

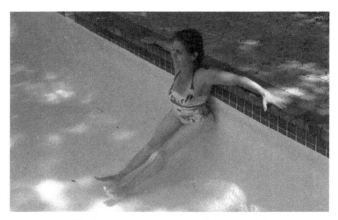

Meditation supported by the pool wall

A moving meditation can also be a no-prop alternative. Borrowing elements from the opening sequence from Ai Chi works as a lovely substitute. Ai Chi is a therapeutic aquatic form that has similarities to Tai Chi and Qi Gong. Invented by Jun Konno, a Japanese Olympic swimming coach, it has been shown to reduce stress and improve the quality of life for people living with diverse conditions such as fibromyalgia and Parkinson's disease.

All movements in Ai Chi are linked to the breath, or Kata in Ai Chi, and should be fluid, relaxed, and graceful. Like any moving meditation, this is about calm, focused awareness, and breath, and less about the form of the movements themselves. You can offer these as a series with multiple repetitions of each pattern, or as individual movements.

Take the lower body form of Goddess pose. Your arms should be straight out of their shoulder sockets, forming a T-shape, palms facing down.

Rotate your palms to face up on an inhale, and rotate your palms to face down on an exhale.

Add in arm movement next. When your palms face down on an exhale, bring your hands down towards your thighs. On an inhale, rotate your palms to face up and bring your palms up towards the surface again, like a bird flapping its wings up and down.

Then switch to bringing your thumbs together on the surface of the water in front on an exhale. Inhale, rotate your palms to face up and on the surface of the water, open your arms back up to a T-shape, like a bird opening and closing its wings.

Next, on an exhale with your palms facing down bring your arms down towards the front of your thighs with shoulder extension. On an inhale, rotate your palms to face up, and bring your palms towards the surface with shoulder flexion.

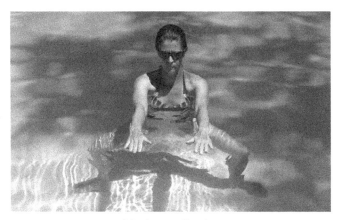

Moving meditation

Continue with adding in an arm cross as you exhale. Instead of bringing your arms straight down, let your arms cross at the elbows and give yourself a hug. Inhale and bring your arms back up to the surface; this time as you exhale, bring your arms down and change the cross so your other arm is on top when you hug yourself.

After several hugs in both directions, open your hands back up to be palms facing under the water. Your elbows are bent with your arms comfortably in front of you. Your palms are gently cupped as if you were holding a ball underwater. On an inhale, visualize the ball you're holding getting bigger as if your lungs were inflating like a beach ball between your hands. As you exhale, the ball deflates, and your hands come closer together. The ball's size relates to the breath, so the ball only inflates as much as your inhale, and deflates to match your exhale. On your final exhale, the ball deflates completely, and your palms touch. Feel the energy between your hands before you leave the meditation.

Floating meditation anecdotes

While the floating meditation part of class is the part where people often say, "Can we just skip to that part at the end?" it's also the part where students and teachers are surprised there are problems.

People bump into each other and parts of the pool—even indoor pools have pumps going, which creates a little bit of current. When people recline into head-back floating meditations, they don't know where they are. The current and/or their own slight movements might push them into each other. If anyone in a class is going to recline, let them know in advance that they might bump into each other or the pool wall/lane dividers, and it's okay, just disconnect and then resume meditating. In an outdoor pool, there might be a considerable breeze. Even people lying down have quite a bit of fetch. The wind will push everyone together at one end of the pool. In an outdoor pool on a windy day, let people know where they might bump into each other or a part of the pool.

Safety becomes a bigger concern. One pool I work at asked us to stop doing the fully reclined meditations. A woman who had been coming to my class had a cardiac event while doing a floating relaxation during open swim hours. The lifeguards didn't respond because they thought she was peacefully floating, as we would in class. She survived, but the ambulance was called later than it would have been otherwise. The moral of the story is to actively watch people while they're meditating and have a defined time limit for your floats.

Both of these points speak to the complexity of a floating meditation environment. People relax and disconnect from what's going on around them in an environment that still has safety concerns. They don't respond to even a slight disruption like brushing fingers in the same way they would in any other part of the class. The most common reaction is one of a bit of disorientation and confusion as people sort themselves out and resume meditating. Occasionally, someone overreacts considerably, and a lot of splashing and thrashing ensues as they get themselves sorted. Help people avoid becoming disorientated at any time by front-loading your directions before meditating and only offer the positions you think are appropriate for your audience. Anticipate safety concerns and adjust accordingly.

What does the research say about floating meditation?

Up to now, research on floating meditation has focused solely on float tanks and the sensory deprivation nature of that experience. A floating meditation as part of a water yoga practice is a more active experience than a float tank meditation, or a traditional seated meditation. Yet, it's more passive than a walking meditation. Like yoga, walking meditation, or Tai Chi, a floating meditation within water yoga can be considered part of the broader category of mindful movement.

Research does show that the physical effects of mindful movement are similar to seated meditation alone. For example, both walking and seated meditation improve the blood sugar levels in people with diabetes. Mindful movement such as Tai Chi, yoga, and seated meditation improves the lung function and mood in COPD patients. Similarly, the mood improvements and stress reduction features of traditional meditation also occur from mindful movement.

Research from float tank meditations shows that they reduce anxiety, stress, and depression, while improving mood. Research into traditional seated meditation has shown similar benefits.

We can only infer if any of these benefits can transfer to a floating meditation in an open pool environment. Further research needs to be done to verify if any of these benefits from similar disciplines apply to a water yoga-based meditation, either as a stand-alone element or as an integral part of a complete water yoga practice.

Facilitating floating meditations is about providing a safe, comfortable environment in the water where people can learn to focus. Offering them at the beginning of a class can create a transition space between the outside world and the yoga environment. Offering them at the end of a class allows people to integrate the class's energetic and physical aspects, in a similar way that a land-based Corpse pose does. Plan your meditations to suit the pool environment you're working in, your students, and your strengths as a teacher.

— Chapter 9 —

How to Sequence Your Water Yoga Classes

What to actually do in the pool is the big question everyone starting a personal water yoga practice faces. That's why they're choosing public classes or private sessions with you, instead of working on their own. As a professional, you know all the parts and how to put them together.

To plan an effective practice for your students, the first thing to figure out is what is the point of the class. It can be a broad physical focus such as effective use of a particular prop, enjoying a specific pose, or smooth transitions. You might choose a therapeutic benefit such as increasing ankle flexibility or supporting knee arthritis by increasing leg strength. It might be emphasizing yoga philosophy such as a specific yoga sutra or one of the less well-known waves such as Pranayama. There are an infinite number of choices so creating an effective class roadmap requires you to choose your destination first.

The process of sequencing is turning one of these areas of focus into a list of actions to take during a class. There are three styles of sequencing (choreography with progressions or regressions in aquatics) that work well for water yoga. A bell curve approach to classes warms students up to a peak pose then winds them down to a floating meditation. An ascendant approach to classes makes everything harder than the last thing to the final challenge, then a sudden shift to meditation. A trekking approach has energetic peaks and valleys throughout the class. It might start with a meditation instead of concluding with one.

Because some teachers find sequencing or creating a lesson plan a challenge, using a template simplifies the process. Instead of a free-for-all roadmap with only a known destination, it lays out consistent markers within the class journey. Using this template, you can overlay any of the three sequencing approaches, adding or moving the meditation to the beginning of the class as needed.

Water yoga class template

1. Introductions
2. Class announcements
3. A big body warm-up
4. Warming up your spine
5. Easier standing poses
6. Harder poses like balance poses
7. Centering/transition poses
8. A floating meditation
9. Closing

All these physical elements highlighted in the template are overlaid with yoga philosophy, breathwork, and concentration practices to support your area of focus.

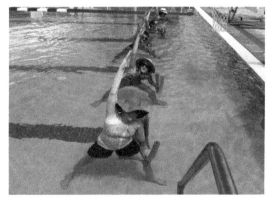

A water yoga class

FAQs about sequencing

How long should people hold each pose?

In the water, holding still like a statue for minutes feels odd, and you get cold. Those are the responses you hear when you literally transfer land yoga into the pool. In a traditional yoga style, such as Iyengar yoga, you might hold an individual pose once for three to five minutes. That discipline focuses on static stretching (a stretch that you hold for longer than 15 seconds).

In water yoga, we can build on the traditions of land yoga and take advantage of the liquid environment by making greater use of dynamic stretching. Research has shown that muscle activity is the same submerged as on land. We can make use of the science of stretching with confidence in the same way in the water. Dynamic stretching takes your muscles and joints through their healthy range of motion. Dynamic stretches are held briefly, less than 15 seconds. Use your breath and Pranayama practices to time your work, rather than a clock. Come into a posture, hold it for three to five breaths, and then come back up to where you started. As an example, starting in Mountain pose, sink down into Chair pose. Hold it three to five breaths, and then come back up to Mountain pose. The average person takes between 12 and 20 breaths per minute, or one breath every three to five seconds. Spend the amount of time in each posture that works for your sequence.

How many times should a student do the pose?

Like most aspects of sequencing, that's a personal decision. I like to offer postures in repetitions of at least three. The first time I give the directions. How to get in and out the pose, the basics. The second time, students are more confident. They can remember to breathe and engage with some of the more subtle aspects of the pose. The third time they can explore the posture more. That means they can settle in internally to notice how the posture makes them feel. You can provide some silence or add variations to challenge students even more.

The number of repetitions, and the length of each repetition, is up to you and your teaching goals. There are many reasons to build up from three repetitions. It can be about wanting more time to explore the posture further, or it might be about feeling cold and wanting more movement. More repetitions might support your application of yoga philosophy or breathwork. You might want to explore the different variations with props and how those make you feel. There can be reasons to add repetitions to only one side and not the other. Notice if there's a relationship between the amount of time you spend in poses and how many times you repeat them.

Should you always come back to Mountain pose between postures?
No. The directions in this book are written to isolate the postures and highlight them individually. You should use transitions that make sense for the sequence you create. That might include using Mountain pose often or only once.

How many poses are in a water yoga class?
A standard water yoga class is 45 minutes long to accommodate the physiological changes that take place in the average pool. Obviously, this can vary depending on the audience and the pool. A young, healthy audience might appreciate a longer one-hour class. If the water temperature is cool, under 80 degrees Fahrenheit, or hot, such as a hot tub, a shorter class would be more appropriate.

In the average 45-minute class I offer 13–15 poses plus a warm-up and floating meditation. In cooler water, I'd offer a faster pace with more arm movements, prop challenges, and more poses during the 45 minutes. If the water is warm, such as a 90-degree Fahrenheit therapy pool, I might offer fewer poses, with slow movements and a long meditation.

Applying the sequencing template
Introduction and announcements
In a class, before launching into directions, I always introduce myself, welcome students to class, and give new people basic orientation facts

such as where the bathrooms are. If I have any class announcements, I try to do those both at the beginning and the end, so more people hear them.

Big body warm-ups

I start every class with some big, whole-body movement. These warm-ups are a transition to getting in the pool and moving. Many people get in the pool with their shoulders scrunched up like earrings and are tiptoeing because it's cool. Warming up gets students comfortable and ready to work. It also lets people chat and have fun before concentrating and getting more serious.

The simplest way to warm up is to walk in the water. When students walk in the water, encourage using the entire sole of the foot. Land on the heel and roll forward towards the toes, then lift the heel into the next stride, just like walking on land. You'll see tiptoeing and bobbing up and down instead. For challenge and variety, students can vary the speed or stride length when walking.

When students seem comfortable, switch to walking backward. The same principles apply in reverse order. Use the full sole of the foot, just like you did when walking forward. You'll see people lean back into the water. You can offer the cues of keeping your front ribs moving back into your spine and your chest lifted. Straighten your leg fully behind you as you reach back with your toes.

Research shows that walking backward is especially beneficial. Walking backward in the water activates the muscles that help support your spine—the erector spinae muscles—more than walking backward on land. These muscles are often weak in people with low back pain. It also helps prevent falls by building the muscles used to lift your lower leg and flex your ankle, both of which get weaker as we age.

As students get comfortable walking backward, suggest varying the speed and stride length. You can combine walking backward and forward to increase the challenge, such as three steps forward, one step backward. This is harder because you're encountering more inertia.

As students get warmer, add in the arms while walking. That can be raising one or both arms overhead. You can move your arms through the water, such as biceps and triceps curls. Pinning one arm to your waist and moving the other in an asymmetrical action increases the challenge.

You can also offer walking sideways in the pool. Cue stepping sideways using the pool edge or a lane divider as a visual marker. Encourage trying to stay parallel to their visual reference. When students run out of room, cue stepping sideways in the other direction. Are everyone's steps the same size when they switch leading legs? Do students stay parallel to the pool wall in one direction but drift forward or backward in the other? These walking variations are more challenging than people think, so they're building body awareness and concentration while they warm up.

Warm-ups can be adaptations of other movements. You can adapt any sport to be a warm-up. Pretend to play: soccer, basketball, ice skating, kayaking or canoeing (with a pool noodle), or a roller derby. You can do dance moves such as a Chubby Checker twist, a grapevine, or square dancing. You can adapt pool games, like sharks and minnows, have lightsaber battles with pool noodles, or hold noodle bicycle races.

Spend the amount of time your students need to feel warmed up. For most people, it's about five minutes. If the water is cooler, they might need a longer or a more vigorous warm-up to feel ready. Have people finish in a part of the pool with level ground where the water comes up to mid-chest height, and come into Mountain pose to start your Asana practice.

Warming up the spine

The next section of a practice is warming up the spine. Warming up the spine involves taking your spine through the six ranges of motion: flexion (folding forward), extension (back arch), twisting in both directions, and a side stretch in both directions. Because spinal flexion happens so often in your daily life, I let that action happen anywhere in the practice, not just the spinal warm-up. The spinal warm-up is where you begin to apply movement with breath, concentration, and yoga philosophy elements. It's your first chance to assess how your students process your cues, so glean information you can use in the rest of the session. Warming up your spine will take anywhere from five to ten minutes of your 45-minute class.

Easier standing poses

If your students are cold or you want to transition directly into Sun Salutations, do that here; otherwise, move into the less challenging standing postures. Less challenging in this context means you're keeping both feet on the ground, and the postures don't require as much balance. They're just as demanding a place to apply yoga philosophy, breathwork, and concentration. The easier poses are ones like Chair, Standing Locust, Down Dog, Warrior II. This section will take five to fifteen minutes of your practice.

Harder poses

Next, you'll challenge your students a bit more with some of the harder aqua yoga poses. These could be the more demanding standing postures, prone/supine postures, or seated poses. You can also make any of your poses harder by using your props and the principles of water to challenge them. Because you're challenging students more with these, remember to cue utilizing the breath, using yoga philosophy, and tips for staying focused. These will take anywhere from five to fifteen minutes of your practice, depending on the effort level you have designed for the session.

Balance postures

Every water yoga practice challenges your balance, but you usually want some postures that are especially considered balance postures. These are the poses that ask students to stand on one leg. These will take approximately five to ten minutes of your practice.

Centering minute

After the concentration and challenge of the balance postures, it's nice to do a few relaxing, stretchy poses before transitioning into floating meditation. This transition time is also a good place to let students check in with themselves and see how they feel. Are there any parts of their body they didn't get to address during the practice? Is there anywhere that worked extra hard and now needs a little stretching out? Allow space for students to get creative with what their bodies need, and encourage doing what feels good. Offer a transition in a grounding posture like Goddess, Chair, or Cat/Cow, to refocus before meditating.

Floating meditation

Your water yoga practice closes with a floating meditation that can take anywhere from three to ten minutes. The time variation accounts for the water temperature, the needs of your students, and the focus of your class. Use the resources in the floating meditation chapter (Chapter 8) that apply to the practice you're designing.

Closing

Public classes end with a closing, thanking people for coming and reiterating any class announcements. For private sessions, I go over the student's homework and take care of scheduling at the end.

Sequencing samples

There are two complete sequences in the book to provide you with both ready-made sequences to teach and examples of how you can assemble a water yoga class. They vary considerably to give you the breadth of what water yoga can offer.

- The Easy One Noodle sequence is a gentle introduction to water yoga. I consider it my go-to sequence when working with new people because it's accessible enough for everyone but flexible enough that I can easily ramp up the challenge dramatically.
- The Core sequence is for everyone who wants to strengthen their core and low back and get more of a workout from water

yoga. It's a great base when you don't have access to equipment or are working with a more athletic population.

These completed practice sequences can also be a sequence learning tool. You can learn to sequence by switching out a pose in these sequences for one you choose. As you feel more confident in sequencing, you insert additional poses or whole sections that you create. These completed sequences follow this same template, so it's easy for you to adjust them.

Easy one noodle water yoga practice

I consider this my go-to sequence when working with new people. As shown below, it's an easy, gentle sequence that's a great introduction to water yoga. It introduces some of the basic poses, has some balance elements, and offers lots of room for adding in the other waves of water yoga. Using tools from this book, you can adjust the difficulty level to suit any audience.

As you're learning to sequence, it's a perfect one to switch some poses out with new ones, or play with the timing until you're ready to create your own sequences from scratch.

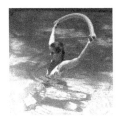

WARRIOR I WALKS – BIG BODY WARM-UP
Step forward two or three steps with one foot. Your knee bends in line with your toes, with the back heel up. Step back to center and repeat on the other side. The noodle can stay in front or can be raised overhead.

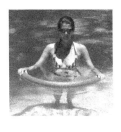

MOUNTAIN POSE – YOGI HOME BASE
Your feet are hip-bone distance apart and parallel. Knees and hips are stacked over your feet. Front ribs draw back towards the spine, and your chest lifts. Shoulder bones are back and down comfortably.

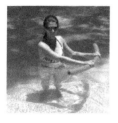

TWISTING MOUNTAIN – SPINAL WARM-UP

From Mountain, with your hands on the noodle, exhale and twist to the right. Inhale back to center, and exhale and twist to the left. Your feet stay in Mountain.

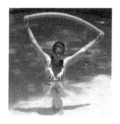

NARROW BASE SIDE STRETCH – SPINAL WARM-UP

In Mountain, bring your feet together or cross your legs. Bring your noodle overhead. Inhale, exhale, lower one edge of the noodle to the water. Inhale to center. Exhale, side stretch the other direction.

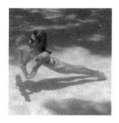

COBRA – SPINAL WARM-UP

In Mountain, with your hands shoulder-distance apart, straighten your arms down against your thighs. Straighten one leg behind you. Point your toes, come onto the top of your foot. Straighten the other leg.

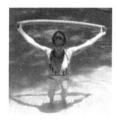

RAINBOW SHOULDER OPENER – EASIER POSE

From Mountain, inhale and lift the noodle overhead. Exhale, spread your shoulders, and lower the noodle behind you with straight arms (okay to let go with one hand), or halfway with bent elbows.

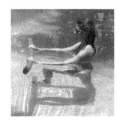

SUNBIRD FLOW — EASIER POSE

From Mountain, inhale, bend one knee, and bring it up, pulling your toes towards your nose. Exhale, straighten your leg out behind you, pointing your toes and setting the tops onto the pool floor.

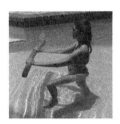

HIP OPENER — EASIER POSE

From the front of Sunbird Flow, pretend you have a paintbrush strapped to your knee and paint lines back and forth. Do both legs and then repeat, pretending your paintbrush is drawing circles now.

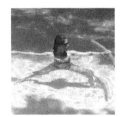

WARRIOR II — EASIER POSE

Come into a wide-legged stance with parallel feet. Turn the toes of one foot out. Bend that knee in line with its toes. Your torso sinks straight down. Your arms are out in a T-shape, with wrists above ankles.

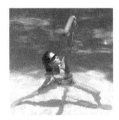

EXALTED WARRIOR — HARDER POSE

From Warrior II, inhale and raise the arm on the bent knee side up overhead. Lower the other hand down to your straight leg. The noodle can be in either hand, and look where it's comfortable.

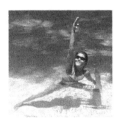

HUMBLE WARRIOR — HARDER POSE

From Warrior II, exhale, and lower the hand on the bent knee side down towards the knee. Raise the other hand up. The noodle can be in either hand, and look where it's comfortable.

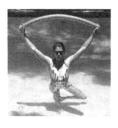

TREE — BALANCE POSE

Stand in Mountain and bend one knee. Pivot the toes to turn the knee out. Connect the sole of the foot to the straight leg, anywhere on the leg except pushing against the knee.

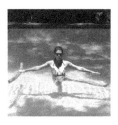

SIDE LEG LIFT — BALANCE POSE

From Tree, straighten the bent knee leg out to the side. Pull your toes to your nose. Hold in Side Leg Lift or flow between Side Leg Lift and Tree. Your hands can be anywhere.

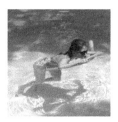

TURTLE — CENTERING POSE

From standing, bring the noodle under your armpits. Lean forwards and bring your feet up off the pool floor. Start with your palms together and knees together and breaststroke over the noodle like a turtle.

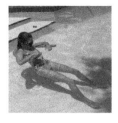

CORPSE — FLOATING MEDITATION

You can simply stop moving in Turtle to do a forward float over your noodle, or move the noodle to behind your shoulders. Enjoy these quiet minutes while letting your body integrate your practice.

Core focused water yoga practice

This sequence takes all the knowledge you've learned and puts it together in a more physically challenging practice which emphasizes the properties of water to challenge your balance and stability. You'll build strength through resisting the water and grounding strongly. Remember, this is a suggested sequence; modify it for your students as needed.

The bulk of the sequence uses no props. You'll need four pool noodles for your floating meditation at the end, as shown here. If you switch that out for a moving meditation the sequence can be done entirely without props. Enjoy the challenge.

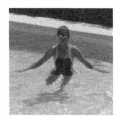

SOCCER PLAYER – BIG BODY WARM-UP
Walk forward around the pool as if you're dribbling a soccer ball. When you feel warm, walk backward by trapping the ball on top, dropping your foot behind the ball, and then kicking it forward.

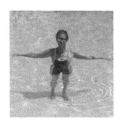

MOUNTAIN POSE – YOGI HOME BASE
Your feet are hip-bone distance apart and parallel. Knees and hips are stacked over your feet. Your chest lifts, shoulder bones are back and down comfortably, and your hands are straight out in a T-position.

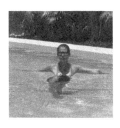

STANDING TWIST – SPINAL WARM-UP
In Mountain, inhale. On an exhale, twist to the right, allowing your spine to twist any amount. Inhale back to center. Exhale as you twist to the left. Your gaze goes where it's comfortable for your neck.

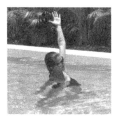

WIDE-LEGGED SIDE STRETCH
– SPINAL WARM-UP
Come into a wide-legged stance with parallel feet. Inhale, raise one arm up overhead. Exhale, drop the other down. Inhale up through center. Exhale, side stretch the other direction.

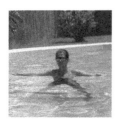

STEPPING STAR — EASIER POSE

In Mountain, with T-position arms, inhale. Exhale, step wide to one side, into wide-legged Mountain. Inhale, step back to Mountain with the same side foot. Repeat the same side several times and then switch.

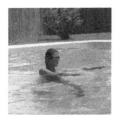

ARM SWEEP STEPPING STAR — EASIER POSE

Repeat Stepping Star, this time sweeping the opposite arm along the surface of the water when you step to the side.

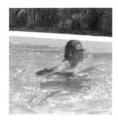

CHAIR — EASIER POSE

In Mountain, with T-shaped arms, inhale in center, exhale, bend your knees. Sink down into an imaginary chair. Concentrate on leaving your feet where they are by weighting the outer edges of them.

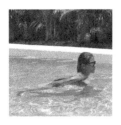

SWINGING CHAIR — EASIER POSE

From Chair, with T-shaped arms, lift one leg and straighten it out in front on an inhale. Tap the heel on the pool floor. Exhale, bring the leg through the center, and straighten the leg behind you, toe tap.

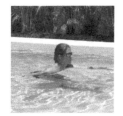

SWINGING CHAIR AND ARM SWEEPS — HARDER POSE

While in Swinging Chair, bring the opposite arm across the surface to be wrist above ankle in front. Open the arm back to a T as the foot comes through the center. Try doing the same side arm and leg next.

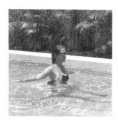

LEG LIFTS — BALANCE POSE

From Mountain, bend one knee. Raise the thigh and straighten your leg out in front of you. Pull the toes back towards your nose and firm your hands against the water for better balance.

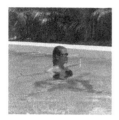

WARRIOR I — EASIER POSE

From Mountain, step straight forward two or three large steps with one foot. The back heel comes up. Exhale, bend the front knee in line with the toes. Your arms are out in a T-shape.

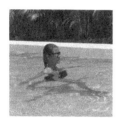

EAGLE RAY WARRIOR I — HARDER POSE

From Warrior I with your arms in a T, keeping your arms straight, exhale, and with palms facing down, bring them down against your hips. Inhale, palms facing up; bring the arms back up to a T on the surface.

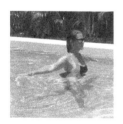

SWINGING LEG LIFT — BALANCE POSE

From Leg Lift, swing the lifted leg out to the side. Toes continue to point up. Hips and gaze face forward. Bring the leg back to the center.

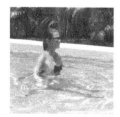

EAGLE RAY SWINGING LEG LIFT — BALANCE POSE

In Swinging Leg Lift, when you're opening your leg out to the side, bring both arms straight down against your hips. Inhale, bring your straight arms back to a T or overhead, and your leg back to center.

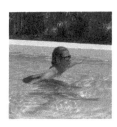

ONE-LEGGED SWINGING CHAIR
– BALANCE POSE

From Chair, straighten one leg in front, toes pointing up. Lift the heel off the pool floor. Swing the lifted leg out to the side. Toes continue to point up, and hips face forward. Bring the leg back to the center.

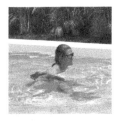

ONE-LEGGED EAGLE RAY – BALANCE POSE

While in One-Legged Swinging Chair, add in bringing both arms straight down against your hips as you take the leg out. Bring your arms back up to the surface as you bring your leg back to the center.

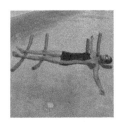

CORPSE POSE – FLOATING MEDITATION

Thread two pool noodles behind your shoulders. Bend your knees and thread more noodles behind your knees. Move one of the shoulder noodles behind your neck, and one of the knee noodles under your ankles.

— Chapter 10 —

Being an Effective Water Yoga Teacher

As water yoga teachers, we want to provide experiences that increase people's sense of agency. Agency is the ability to make things happen for yourself. To have survived to adulthood, you have to have had enough agency to meet your basic needs; foods, shelter, and so on. To be happy, you need to apply that agency to more than the basics of survival.

A water yoga class tries to foster an environment that allows for safe exploration. We want people to feel safe to try new things and to find out new things about themselves also. We are facilitators of learning experiences that increase self-actualization. As such, we need good communication skills to provide positive experiences using the tools of water yoga.

A simple acronym highlights the essential verbal skills you need to be a great water yoga teacher: SWIM.

S: Succinct

Don't use three words if you can use one. Cueing is not Shakespeare. Use descriptive, active phrases with plenty of action verbs. "Allow the arms to float up through the water, break the surface, and rise up overhead" is a lot. Everyone can hear and comprehend, "Raise your arms up." Use active, specific language rather than vague, passive phrasing.

W: Welcoming

Ahimsa is the first principle in yoga. All your students will always be doing more things right than they are doing wrong. Focus on the positive and compliment what's working. Offer suggestions for improvement based on your students' needs.

I: Important

Sequentially dole out information. Safety is paramount, so always lead with that. Then move into specific directions. Leave the fluff until the end if there's time. Use the iceberg principle. There's always more to say, but start with what gets the job done and expand from there.

M: Meaningful

Meet your students where they are. You would never tell a group of seniors at their first yoga class to "Perform all your postures today with the principles of Sthira and Sukha, so your Vrittis don't get stuck in your Samskaras." You'd say, "You're here to move past your bad habits. Let's improve your balance and build some strength with Warrior II pose. Firmly ground your feet into the pool floor, bend your leading knee, and use your breath to raise your arms up."

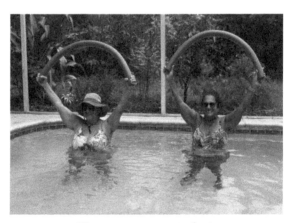

Happy water yoga students

Practical teaching considerations

- How much you physically demonstrate is up to you. Remember to demonstrate at the intensity level where most of your students are performing. Demonstrate the options starting with those of least intensity to those of most intensity, but then settle back down into the mid-range where most of your students are. Don't demonstrate at such an intensity that none of your students can participate.

- When teaching from the pool deck or when facing your students, it makes sense to mirror them. When teaching in the round, such as in the pool, demonstrate the same side.

- When teaching in the water, people can't see your feet. You can use your hands as proxy feet. Flat palms would represent the soles of the feet on the pool floor. Point the fingers down and bend your wrist to mimic bringing the toes to the pool floor, and so on. Sometimes it makes sense to bring your toes out of the water to show positioning. For example, in Side Leg Lift pose, you don't want to demonstrate with your leg on the surface of the water unless it's relevant to your students. Still, you could bring your toes up momentarily to show where they are in relation to your torso.

- With the water's surface dividing people's bodies in half, there can be a tendency to focus on where people are looking and what their arms are doing in the pool. Water yoga teaching is the same as mat yoga in that you offer cues and feedback starting from the base and working up. Once a student's base is solid and reflects where it should be, give your cues from there. The same pattern follows when offering feedback. If someone is twisting the wrong way in a class, make suggestions starting at the base and work up. In water yoga, the base of postures is most likely to be your feet, but it can be your bum or your back or belly. Train yourself to look at the base of support first, and everything flows from there.

- When students are struggling with buoyancy, make suggestions proximally to distally. Engaging their core muscles will be a more effective stabilizer than tightening their grip on a pool noodle.
- It's hard to hear in pool environments. Don't use a "yoga voice." A yoga voice is soft and lilting. If you saw the Harry Potter movies, Luna Lovegood used a yoga voice. Luna would be a lovely meditation teacher in a calm and quiet yoga studio. She wouldn't be effective in a busy pool.
- If you struggle with speaking loudly or your voice is naturally high-pitched, a sound system will really help. Ask the facility you teach at if you can use theirs, or buy a portable one for yourself.
- Hands-on assists are not practical in the pool. You're either on the pool deck or can't wade through the water fast enough to get to each student at the relevant moment.
- As water yoga teachers, remember yoga philosophy: practice Ahimsa and acknowledge what's working for your students before offering suggestions for improvement.

Teaching mixed-level classes

The odds are that every public class you teach will be a mixed-level class. This means that you'll have the full spectrum of experience with yoga and aquatics, from total newbies to some with experience. Unless they've been coming to your classes, it's rare for a student to have prior experience with water yoga. These are tips for adjusting poses to help everyone to be successful. Always start with the most accessible option. Add in choices until everyone has something to choose from that works for them. That doesn't mean every pose begins at the absolute easiest level. That means every pose you offer starts at the place where everyone can do it. A group of more advanced students will begin at an overall harder level. However, don't label them "easiest/best/fullest." Everyone is there to do their personal best. They're just choosing the "options and variations" that best suit their needs.

Using Dancer's pose as an example of this accessible approach

Option number one: Start with Standing Locust pose.

Option number two: Add lifting the heel towards the bum on the back leg in Standing Locust pose to add standing on one leg.

Option number three: Repeat the heel towards the bum on an inhale, and lower the foot back down to the pool floor on an exhale.

Option number four: Add in a transverse arm sweep by swinging the hand on the surface of the water on the same side as the raised leg back on the inhale. On the exhale, when you lower the foot, return the arm to in front of you.

Option number five: Hold the foot with the hand on the same side.

Option number six: While holding the foot, hinge forward in the standing leg hip.

Option number seven: Reach back with the other hand and hold the foot with both hands.

Option number eight: Alternate which hand holds the foot dynamically as a transverse arm sweep. Bring the alternating hands forward and back to your foot, timed to your breath.

Option number nine: Come to tiptoes on the standing leg in any of these variations.

These nine options break one posture down into a full practice spectrum from very easy to very demanding. You can apply the techniques of making poses easier and harder to any pose, so that each student in your class will always be able to choose the appropriate level to work at.

Adding choices to affect the challenge in postures
Ways to make postures easier

- Reduce the length of time in the pose.
- Reduce the number of repetitions.
- Use the pool steps or wall for support.
- Adjust your base (this might mean wider or narrower, depending on the posture).
- Reduce the depth of the stance (don't bend the knees as much to reduce the load or joint demand).
- Keep the toes on the floor instead of lifting the leg for one-legged postures.
- Use a prop for support, depending on the prop and pose.
- Keep the arms open on the surface of the water for support.

Ways to make postures harder

- Add asymmetry (one side of the body does something different from the other in symmetrical poses).
- Add contralateral movements (diagonal arms and legs).
- Add ipsilateral movements (movement on the same side of the body).
- Use multiple planes of movement (instead of both arms and legs moving in the sagittal plane, legs move in the sagittal, and arms move in the coronal).
- Change the movement planes to be non-traditional yoga planes, such as transverse arm movements in Warrior I.
- Change the breath pattern. Instead of inhaling on arms up, exhale on arms up, for example.
- Add water resistance by moving the limbs.
- Move the arms above the water, while the legs move below. The water's resistance on only half the body creates a timing challenge.

- Vary the timing of movements, such as moving the arms with one breath, but the legs with two.
- Take one-legged postures to the tiptoes.
- Instead of a fixed focal point, follow a moving limb with the eyes.
- Use a prop to reinforce these actions or add another challenge.

Your teachings should reflect you

What is your definition of yoga?

What you offer as a teacher should reflect your thoughts on water yoga. Your language choices, what you demo, which aspects of the practice you emphasize should all reflect your approach to yoga. For example, the way you teach each pose should follow your definition of what the pose is about. Putting this into practice, what do you believe the point of Tree pose is?

- Is it a balance posture?
- Is it about external hip rotation?
- Is it about raising the arms overhead in shoulder flexion and forming a mudra with the hands to create branches?
- Is it the perfect place to challenge yourself with Tapas?
- Is it the ideal physical form to complement a Pranayama practice?

How you describe the pose to students should reflect what you believe the pose to be about. If you're emphasizing balance, it will be more important for your students to stand on one leg than to turn their hip out and leave their toes on the pool floor.

If you want water yoga to look exactly like land yoga, you'll teach the same as on land. Your sequences would emphasize postures that look exactly the same in the water and on land, like Triangle pose. If you emphasize movement over forms, your water yoga practice will look very different from land yoga by exploiting the physics of exercising in the water. How much creativity and deviation from traditional land yoga you're comfortable with is up to you.

You want your students to own their practice

The highest compliment our students can give us is to not need us anymore because they have developed a personal water yoga practice. Their sense of agency regarding water yoga has become strong enough that they can take full ownership of their own program. For students looking to move in that direction, here are some suggestions on transitioning to a personal practice:

- Add a yoga pose to the beginning or end of the existing pool time. Increase the number gradually.
- Read a yoga philosophy book.
- Apply breathwork practices to an aqua aerobics class.
- Book a package of private sessions with the goal of moving to a personal practice.
- Start a once per week meditation practice outside class.
- Start a reflection journal to record thoughts about water yoga practice.
- Get together outside class to learn from other students.

One of the most valuable lessons to remember as a teacher is that we are all students first. To teach water yoga, you need a personal water yoga practice. Spend some time with the resources in the book to develop your own practice before you try teaching these ideas publicly. Notice how the different pose variations and options from the other seven limbs of yoga impact you personally day to day, in various water depths, and with different props. As you begin to teach, be a student of teaching water yoga. Notice how your teachings are received and hone and refine your craft from the feedback you receive. As you get comfortable teaching, continue to explore aspects of the craft that are beyond this book's scope.

— Chapter 11 —

Integrating Water Science and Yoga Systems in Water Yoga

Water yoga is yoga, and can't be divorced from that discipline any more than you can ignore that it happens in water. As a blended discipline, it also straddles the world of science. These disciplines have more in common than you might think, and each impacts your students' practice and bodies in tangible ways. The Chakras' energetic features, the philosophical aspects of the elements in yoga, and the physics and properties of water synergistically create an environment where people can experience profound personal change.

Chakra means wheel, and these are energy centers corresponding to anatomical regions in your body. The energy they contain helps those parts of your body function efficiently, as well as helps you regulate your energetic and emotional states. There are seven Chakras in your body: Root, Sacral, Solar Plexus, Heart, Throat, Third Eye, and Crown.

The elements in yoga are a philosophical idea that structures the world around us. The original yogis didn't have modern science to organize the world, but they had the power of observation. Categorizing the world into elements gives us a way to see ourselves in the bigger picture of nature and the universe. While there are seven Chakras in yoga, there are only five elements: Earth, Water, Fire, Air, and Ether.

The physics of movement in water is critical to know as a water yoga professional because it's central to the practice. The water is an essential part of water yoga. You have to have it. You have to move through it. Unlike air, you probably don't have a lifetime of experience moving through the water to "wing it" as a teacher. Some of these ideas might not be instinctual, so you need a working knowledge of them to keep your students safe, and provide them with an appropriate level of challenge. These seven aquatic principles are the most impactful to water yoga practice: buoyancy, center of gravity versus center of buoyancy, viscosity, hydrostatic pressure, surface tension, knowledge of the anatomical planes, and inertia.

Just like the physical aspects of yoga, we're starting at the base and our physical foundation, and working up towards our spiritual awareness as we talk about these ideas. The Chakras and elements are associated with distinct parts of your body. However, the physics of water applies to all of you, just not necessarily equally everywhere. Surface tension will affect your Heart and Throat Chakras the most because that's where the surface tension happens. Viscosity, however, impacts everything you have underwater. I've associated viscosity with building strength and confidence with the Solar Plexus Chakra and the Fire element. It still applies to all the other Chakras and elements. When you're done with this chapter, leave the Chakras and elements in the order they're listed here and think about how you would interpret the impact of the aquatic principles if you paired them differently.

Each of these sections has a teaching sample to see how these ideas can be interpreted in a practical way. As a teacher, you'll want to create your own original scripts that highlight your interpretation of these ideas also.

The base of your spine

Your Root Chakra (Muladhara Chakra) is located at the base of your spine. It correlates to feeling grounded and safe. You use your Root Chakra when making decisions about survival issues like money and food.

The Earth element is about the literal ground and physicality of the soil. But it's also about everything solid and tangible. Your bones and physical self correspond to the Earth element. The Earth element speaks to the physical benefits your students might receive from a practice.

Archimedes' principle of buoyancy states that the loss of weight you experience in the water equals the weight of the fluid you are displacing. Your density impacts your buoyancy. More muscular people are denser; therefore, they sink because they displace less water. A person with more body fat floats because they displace more water.

The average person is offloading half their weight at their belly button, 70 percent at mid-chest height, and 90 percent when submerged to their neck. For water yoga, practicing at mid-chest height is ideal. Very buoyant people benefit from shallower water while they learn to ground themselves.

When people are buoyant in the water, they feel less grounded and attached to the earth. For people who are afraid of the water, this is especially scary and puts them in touch with their root survival instincts. Be patient with people who are fearful of the water. Everyone learns to ground themselves better through water yoga, and this is one of the chief physical benefits of the practice.

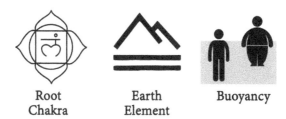

| | Root Chakra | Earth Element | Buoyancy |

Teaching idea

Kelp plants attach themselves firmly to the ocean floor. That connection to the earth is vital to their survival. They are not free-floating algae, and need to be tethered to the Earth element. Like you, they use the buoyancy of the water to support their leaves. The water lets the leaves fan out and receive the sun's rays. Firmly ground into your feet, like the holdfast qualities of Pacific kelp. Reach out with your arms on the surface of the water. Feel the water support your arms. Press into your firm hold on the bottom of the pool. Feel that solidity up your legs into the base of your spine at the Root Chakra. Reach up through the crown of your head towards the sun. Feel the buoyancy provided by the water. Feel the firm, safe connection your feet give you. Be grounded, but tall and flexible like kelp.

Your pelvis

Your Sacral Chakra (Svadhisthana Chakra) is located in your lower abdomen, a couple inches below your belly button. It relates to regulating your feelings and emotions and responding to the emotions of those around you. You use your Sacral Chakra to be creative and control sexual energy.

The Water element corresponds to all liquids. It relates to all the fluids in your body. Your body is naturally up to 60 percent water. Before you were born, you lived in water inside your mother. It was once your home element. Returning to the water can remind you of the emotional state of being deeply connected with another. It's an opportunity to use the water's physical aspects to help buoy and regulate your emotional states.

For most people, the feet and legs tend to sink. That pulls your torso into the water from the bum, while your chest area wants to float. Your center of gravity is located low in your torso around your belly button. Your center of buoyancy is up in your chest. To think about the relationship between your center of gravity versus buoyancy, think of a boat with a crow's nest at the top of the mast. If it's a small boat and a person climbs into that basket and throws themselves side to side, the boat will start to pitch. The same idea applies in water yoga. Think of the weight displacement of a person with poor posture who carries their head forward. That person's center of gravity and buoyancy has shifted forward, making it harder for them to balance while standing.

Conversely, think of a large pear-shaped woman with a very ample behind. Because of the physics of buoyancy, her center of gravity and buoyancy have flipped. Pretend she's seated on a noodle and swaying her feet back and forth a bit. Her ample bum is her center of buoyancy, which is going to float. Her head and chest area is her center of gravity and is going to sink. It's as if the crow's nest has been flipped upside down, and the movement of her feet is going to drive her head underwater. That becomes a safety hazard fast if her head gets in the water with her feet on the surface, and she doesn't know what to do.

Sacral
Chakra

Water
Element

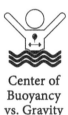
Center of
Buoyancy
vs. Gravity

Teaching idea with a kickboard

Notice that your kickboard has a rounded end and a flat end. Tuck the flat end against the back of your knees. While holding on to the kickboard with both hands, sit back on the kickboard. Your knees are bent and your feet are below you, as if you're seated on a floating chair. The kickboard will support you but it needs to be parallel to the pool floor. That keeps your center of buoyancy over your center of gravity. Bring your awareness down into your Sacral Chakra so you can maintain your balance. Stay seated on the kickboard. Bend and straighten your legs one at a time. Notice how you're feeling. If you're feeling confident, can you let go of the kickboard with one hand? Keep control of your kickboard. Your neighbor is not going to be happy with you if it comes shooting out, so maybe continue to hold on to it with one hand. This is a creative adaptation of Staff pose, making use of the element of Water. What would be fun to do with both your hands—keep them on the surface, move them through the water? Can you move both your hands and legs at the same time? Anything else you want to try?

- Whenever you're doing postures seated on a kickboard, make sure your students are spread out and can control their kickboards. Kickboards can pop out of the water quickly, and with a lot of force.

Your lower organs

Your Solar Plexus Chakra (Manipura Chakra) is located in the upper abdomen around your stomach. It relates to your confidence and feelings of agency in your life. When you have butterflies in your stomach because you're nervous, that's your Solar Plexus Chakra needing support.

The Fire element is about transformation. You use heat and energy to create something else. Think of the expression, "fire in your belly." You're supercharged and ready to go. The Fire element tells you to eat, drink, and sleep, so you're fueled for the next big thing.

The dynamic, moving postures we do in water yoga stoke the Fire element. We use the water's viscosity and density to amplify the postural elements of water yoga. We're getting stronger and more capable in the water so we can meet challenges with courage and confidence when we're out of the water.

Viscosity is the friction between liquid or gas molecules that causes them to stick together and to you. Water is more viscous than air, and honey is more viscous than water. The friction between molecules is partly what makes movement harder underwater than on land. You can use this principle to help keep people warm, challenge their balance, and increase their strength during water yoga.

Solar Plexus   Fire   Viscosity
Chakra   Element

Teaching idea with two pool noodles

You're going to build some heat and confidence by taking Plank pose through into Reverse Plank pose as a flow. For Plank pose, start in Mountain pose with one noodle centered in each hand. Bring the noodles down alongside your legs, thumbs against your outer thighs with straight arms. Keeping your arms straight and the noodles loaded, step back with one leg. Anchor the tips of the toes to the pool floor and straighten your leg. Bend the other knee and step back with that leg. You're now on all ten toes with straight legs in Plank pose. Be one long line from the crown of your head reaching back to your heels. Your tummy and hips are not sagging down towards the pool floor. Reach back into your heels with confidence and intent. You've got this.

To come into Reverse Plank pose, bend both knees and draw them up towards your hands. Keep your knees and feet together while you bring them up. Your arms are still straight and shoulder-distance apart. You're in a floating Chair pose. The noodles will hold you up. Still keeping your knees and feet together, shoot your legs out in front of you. Attach the soles of both feet to the pool floor in front of you. Your arms are still straight and shoulder-distance apart. Your hands will shift forward and back slightly as you move through the two poses. Reach down into your Sacral Chakra and keep your belly and hips lifted in Reverse Plank pose. Reverse Plank can be harder. Can you find your confidence again?

Bend your knees, keep the knees and feet together as you draw your legs back up into your suspended Chair pose. Shoot both your feet back behind you into Plank pose. Continue this flow for five more rounds. Notice how much resistance you feel from the water. As you've done this a couple of times, notice that you're getting warmer. It's getting easier. You're feeling more comfortable doing it even as it's getting to be more work. You're stoking the Fire element and building some heat and confidence. When you're done, notice how you feel—limber, strong, stable. You're ready for the next thing. Let's do it.

Your heart

Your Heart Chakra (Anahata Chakra) is located over your heart. That's the ideal place for the waterline to be on your body when you practice water yoga. The Heart Chakra marks the transition from the material, bodily energies to the spiritual energies. It is linked to your ability to give and receive love.

The Air element is everything that's gas. It is the life force, the energy, the Prana in your body. You circulate your energy with your breath. That's why breath practices are called "Prana"yama. Pranayama and breath practices use the Air element to revitalize yourself.

Air is yoga. Jivana Heyman, the founder of Accessible Yoga, likes to say, "If you have a body, and you can breathe, you can do yoga." The yoga sutras only mention one yoga pose, a seated position, but they mention breathing dozens of times. It's the job of your heart to move that oxygenated, energy-rich, Prana-filled blood around. If the hydrostatic pressure makes that job easier, it gives you more energy to engage with the heart's symbolic task—to love and care for yourself and others.

Hydrostatic pressure is the pressure exerted on a submerged body by water molecules. Water is 800 times denser than air. It's why it feels as if you've climbed into a tight sock squeezing in on you when you get in the water. The hydrostatic pressure reduces blood pooling in your feet, and swelling in general. More blood up in your torso makes your heart more efficient. The hydrostatic pressure makes breathing harder, so it has a significant impact on Pranayama practices. It also makes your kidneys more efficient, which is why you need to use the bathroom so soon after being in the pool.

Heart
Chakra

Air
Element

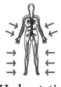

Hydrostatic
Pressure

Teaching idea

In Mountain pose, bring your hands comfortably to the surface of the water. To warm up, you're going to move some energy around your body. Inhale in the center, feel your chest and ribs expand against the water. Exhale while twisting any amount to the right. When you run out of breath, or your spine moves as much as it wants, inhale back to the center. Exhale, pause and feel the hydrostatic pressure of the water squeeze the carbon dioxide out of you. Inhale, feel how the pressure makes it a little harder to breathe. Exhale while you twist any amount to the left. Inhale back to the center.

As you breathe this time, notice the energy coming into your body with each inhale. As you exhale and twist to the right, notice the relaxation and the ease from your breath. Inhaling back to the center, you're using the Air element to send energy or Prana throughout your body. Inhale and exhale, twist to the left. Inhale back to the center.

Do this three more times in each direction. As you inhale and exhale, feel the Prana move through your body. You're twisting through the center of your chest where your Heart Chakra is. Your heart is going to nourish you throughout class today. Feel that energy come into you, and energize your heart. Feel the love and self-care in every exhale. Maintain this connection between your breath and loving energy as you practice today.

Your throat

Your Throat Chakra (Vishuddha Chakra) resides over your throat. It's linked to your ability to communicate and express your truth. When you have an idea you need to express, you say, "What's rising to the surface," or "bubbling up."

The Ether element is space. It represents the plane of open spaciousness that makes connecting with a higher power possible. It's what's between you and whatever else is out there. Space is responsible for your connection with other people. You're not shouting out into the empty ether. People, and if you're religiously observant, a higher power, are right next to you, ready to receive what you have to say.

We can use the Ether element to create a connection with others in water yoga classes. Your students practice water yoga in their own bodies, but they come to class to practice in a community. Just as water molecules are drawn together through surface tension, people are drawn together. They want to communicate across the space between them, and form friendships and connections.

Surface tension is the attractive force between the surface molecules of a fluid. This creates the "skin" on the surface of a liquid. Because of surface tension (combined with the sudden change in viscosity), it is more effort to move a limb through the water's surface than to leave it entirely above, or below, the water.

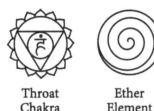

| Throat Chakra | Ether Element | Surface Tension |

Teaching idea

From Mountain pose, step wide with both feet. Wider than shoulder-distance but still comfortable for you. Bring your feet back to parallel. Feel the wide space between your legs making you stable. That's the Ether element surrounding you. Your hands are on the surface of the water, palms facing up. We're going to do a group chant today. You're going to chant, "Yoga makes me strong." Take an inhale and exhale in preparation. Inhale and lift your arms up into a big V shape. It's V for victory. Really loud, everybody says, "Yoga makes me strong." Lower your arms back to the surface. Again, inhale big V shape. "Yoga makes me strong." This time drop your arms down alongside your thighs. Inhale, bring your palms up through the surface of the water overhead into a V. Loud now, you just have to apply a lot of force to break the surface tension of the water. "Yoga makes me strong." Last time, lower the arms down alongside your legs. Your Throat Chakra is warmed up now so make sure they can hear you inside the sauna. See if we can get them to join us next time. Inhale and bring your arms through the water, up overhead into a big, strong V. Together, "Yoga makes me strong." Notice how you're all smiling. Because you're all building strength and having a good time together.

Your head

Your Third Eye Chakra (Ajna Chakra) is located between your eyes and governs intuition and knowledge. Your Third Eye is commonly expressed as what allows you to see. Not see with your eyes, but with wisdom.

As there is no element in yoga associated with the Third Eye Chakra, it provides an opportunity to use your intellect, curiosity, and inner wisdom to integrate all the elements into your practice. While we're discussing these ideas as concrete thoughts, in your body they're not isolated. They can affect you just in certain areas, but more likely, you're noticing them as integrated parts of the totality of your practice.

Within the discipline of anatomy, your body is divided into three movement planes; sagittal, coronal/frontal, and transverse. The sagittal plane divides your body into left and right halves with an imaginary line down your midline. The coronal plane is perpendicular to the sagittal, and imaginarily divides your body in half from front to back. The transverse plane imaginarily cuts you in half from top to bottom. When you describe a movement, the movement happens in the plane that the moving body part is parallel to. For example, movement in the sagittal plane happens parallel to a yoga mat's outside edges, like raising your arms in Warrior I pose. In the coronal plane, movement happens as if you were standing in a doorframe, like hinging in your hip and raising your top arm in Half Moon pose. In the transverse plane, movement happens parallel to the ground, like looking back over your shoulder in a spinal twist.

Land yoga takes place on a rectangular mat. The shape of that mat has constricted many yoga movements to mostly the sagittal plane. In the pool, there is no mat. You're free to do yoga in any direction. That allows you to move in previously unexplored ways. It enables you to be creative with your interpretation of traditional postures. You can apply your intuition and inner wisdom to your practice without any fear of slipping, or deviating from prescribed forms because you stepped off your rectangle. Three hundred and sixty degrees of movement are now available to you.

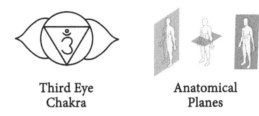

Third Eye
Chakra

Anatomical
Planes

Teaching idea

From Mountain pose, bend your knees, and sink straight down into an imaginary chair. Pretend your Chair pose is the center of a clock face. The center of the clock is right between your feet. Your arms can be anywhere. Staying in your Chair pose, straighten your right leg out in front of you. Set the heel of the right leg on the pool floor at 12:00. Keeping the right heel on the pool floor, sweep the right leg out to the side through to 3:00. At 3:00, your ankle will need to pivot so you're on your right toes. You'll end up at 6:00 with your right leg straight out behind you on your tiptoes. The rest of your body stays in Chair pose. You have just swept your right leg through the transverse plane. Bring it up back to Chair pose in the center through the sagittal plane. Do the same thing on the left side. Using your Third Eye Chakra and your proprioceptive skills, you don't need to watch your left leg come in front, sweep to 3:00, and finish at 6:00.

Come back into Chair pose. Using all the movement planes and your body awareness, add in your arms. Open your arms straight out to the sides in a T-shape. Pivot your wrists so your thumbs face up to the sky. Straighten your right leg out in front to 12:00. As you sweep your right leg around to 3:00, bring both arms straight up overhead, thumbs and forefingers touching in a triangle. That's moving through the coronal plane. As you rotate your ankle around and sweep your toe to 6:00, bring your arms back down into a T. Great job on the body awareness and coordination. Bring the right leg back to Chair pose. Now do the same thing on the other side.

Straighten your left leg out in front to 12:00. This is the sagittal plane. As you sweep your left leg on the heel around to 9:00 in the transverse plane, bring both arms straight up overhead in the coronal plane. As you rotate your ankle around and sweep your toe to 6:00 in the transverse plane, bring your arms back down into a T in the coronal plane. Bring your left leg back to Chair pose through the sagittal plane and come back up to standing.

Again, do this one more time on each side. This is a lot of coordination. Your Third Eye Chakra's got you covered. You can do it. Swing the right leg in front. Sweep it to the side as you move your arms up and down. Back to the center. See, no headaches. Last time on the left. Swing the left leg in front. Sweep it to the side as you raise and lower your arms. Back to the center and stand up. Take a little wiggle to work that out.

- Vary this to emphasize different planes of movement. For example, the leg can go forward and back between 12:00 and 6:00 on your imaginary clockface in the sagittal plane. The arms can sweep the surface of the water between 12:00–3:00 and 12:00–9:00 respectively, in the transverse plane.

The top of your body

Your Crown Chakra (Sahasrara Chakra) is located at the crown of your head. It's the most spiritual of the Chakras and linked to your consciousness and connection to a higher power. Just as you encounter inertia in the pool in stages, depending on what you're doing, you can layer on the skills you have developed through applying the concepts from the previous Chakras and elements to support you in a spiritual practice.

It takes effort to overcome inertia. When there's greater resistance, it takes even more effort. If you're going to develop a spiritual practice, it takes overcoming the inertia of this physical realm. It takes dedicated practice despite all the distractions of everyday life. Building strength through battling inertia in the water can help you build the dedication required for a consistent spiritual practice.

You've probably heard inertia defined as: an object at rest tends to stay at rest, and an object in motion tends to stay in motion. In water, there are actually three kinds of inertia your body experiences: limb, whole body, and water.

Limb inertia: Because of the water's resistance, it takes more muscular effort to start a movement when submerged. Also, because of the water's greater resistance, it takes less effort to stop a movement than it does in air. Inertia helps you build strength faster, while reducing injury risk, compared to land exercise. If you bend your elbow to bring your hand to your shoulder, your biceps muscle encounters greater resistance when submerged than it does on land. If any pain occurs during that movement, the water counteracts your momentum. Your arm stops moving faster, and therefore the pain stops faster.

Whole body inertia: In water, it takes more effort to start, change direction, or stop your whole body compared to moving through the air. Think of how much surface area your body has when moving. This can be used to help keep people warm or increase the challenge during water yoga.

Water inertia: Think of your students in a single-file line walking in the same direction in the water during a water yoga class. If they suddenly all turned around to walk the other way, they'd encounter the current they created (the water's inertia). Again, this principle can be used both to keep people warm and to increase the challenge during classes.

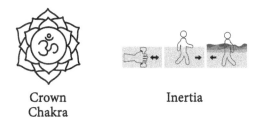

Crown
Chakra

Inertia

Teaching idea

You're going to finish class today with a moving meditation. Everyone comes into a circle, facing the back of the person in front of you. Make the circle large enough that you have enough space between you and the next person—at least three feet. You're going to walk forward. You'll need to adjust your pace to match the pace of the person in front of you. You don't want to walk up on top of them. Everyone is walking the same speed. Notice how hard it is to keep your balance while you're walking, and keep pace with everyone else in the circle. All the distractions of your everyday life have dropped away, haven't they? Use this in your meditation today. If you feel yourself getting drawn out of the pool by a noise, or something going on inside your head, bring your awareness back to stabilizing your feet, the water against your body, the physical act of walking.

Now everyone's going to spin 180 degrees and walk in the other direction. Woah! That got hard, didn't it? That's the water's inertia. Your whole body is encountering the current you all just made. Notice as you keep walking this direction, it's getting easier because you're overcoming the inertia. It's the same thing in your meditation. You're trying to connect with and soothe your consciousness, and maybe connect with something larger than yourself and a higher power. Your Crown Chakra is at the top of your head. It didn't feel the inertia of the water like the rest of you did. It's the same thing in your meditation—you make it harder on yourself than it has to be by getting buffeted by the forces around you.

Spin around one more time. Now you know it's coming. You can deal with the inertia. You've got this. You can stay connected and focused in your practice. You're disciplined. And wherever you are, stop. Feel the water continuing to move against you for a moment. And widen your stance to be comfortable, with bent knees. The water comes up to your neck. Bring your arms under the water and move them back and forth. Now you've got the inertia of your arms moving through the water. But you know how to deal with it, you've got the discipline. You're not letting the water toss you around. And gently let your arms become still and float to the surface of the water. If you want to close your eyes, gently close them. If you'd rather leave them open, bring your gaze to the surface of the water and let your eyelids be heavy.

Connect with your Crown Chakra again. Stay calmly centered inside yourself and your consciousness. There's nothing you need to think about. There's nowhere you need to go. You're just being. At one with yourself and the universe.

As a water yoga teacher, depending on your perspective, you might have an easier time connecting with the scientific, philosophical, or energetic aspects of water and yoga. However, as teachers, we're serving our students who will connect with these ideas differently. A well-rounded teacher is informed by all these ideas and presents the practice in its totality. By offering all aspects of the practice, you'll be able to serve your students with the ideas that resonate with them.

Chapter 12

Water Yoga through the Ages and Stages

There are special considerations you need to make for certain populations who come to water yoga. However, rather than think of water yoga as serving people who live with a specific health condition, it's helpful to use a "people first" perspective. Many health conditions can affect people at any age. Women experience pregnancy as a normal part of life, and getting old is a privilege we all hope to receive. These are ideas to serve people of different ages, and at different stages of their lives.

There's a historical timeline to the foundational texts of yoga. The sutras were the first texts, followed by the Vedas and then others. The principles in the Vedas build on the foundation of the sutras, especially in regards to yoga philosophy. Within the Vedic tradition of yoga, there are four stages, or Ashramas, in our lives.

- Student, or Brahmacharya, where we focus on learning life skills and good values to grow up to be functional, successful, and happy adults.
- Householder, or Grihastha, where we focus on our jobs and families.
- Retiree, or Vanaprastha, where we focus less on material distractions and more on helping our kids raise their kids. Also, our own spiritual path.

- Renunciate, or Sannyas, where we focus entirely on spiritual development rather than worldly matters.

Water yoga can help people in different ways as they go through these stages in their life. For example, water yoga for kids should focus on fun, developing gross motor skills, teamwork, and cooperation. Water yoga for pregnancy should help women make the transition from being independent adults to raising other humans. Retirees need water yoga to help with the challenges of aging bodies and shifting priorities. As they move into the Renunciate stage, some people use water yoga as part of their spiritual practice.

This overlaps very well with how most aquatics classes are structured as well. Many pools offer swimming classes for kids, fitness classes geared towards pregnant women, and a host of programs for seniors. This is so that students get their needs met in a cohort of similar people. Homogeneous cohorts also make these ideas easier to implement than mixed-age classes.

These are suggestions for how to help people as they navigate these various life stages. On average, the following conditions affect people at certain ages and stages. However, that isn't always the case. Arthritis, for example, can affect people at any age. All students need to practice Svadhyaya to work within the balance of Ahimsa and Tapas for them as individuals. For anyone with a health challenge, this is even more important. Encourage each student to practice at their own level. As a teacher, keep in mind best practices for specific conditions.

While the stages are established within the structure of yoga, I'm only covering a few conditions within the large number of diagnoses people face. These conditions included are common within the population of people who come to aquatics classes. If your students live with other conditions and you don't have experience with those, that's okay. The student is always the expert on their own body, so just clarify, they need to pay attention to their own bodies and do what's best for them during class. You can always research other conditions, do continuing education, or reach out to fellow professionals for advice on any diagnoses not included here.

Every student with a health diagnosis should clear their exercise program with their healthcare provider before exercising. Remember, your scope of practice is to provide water yoga instruction. This information is provided to help you meet student needs appropriately, not for the diagnosis or treatment of any condition by you. As water yoga teachers, we don't treat any particular disease. However, we can offer water yoga in concert with best practices for people who live with certain conditions. We stay in our scope of practice, and our students receive the greatest benefits.

Student/Brahmacharya stage
Water yoga for kids

I think of water yoga for kids as creating fun and calm during a hurricane. Kids love to be in the pool, diving and splashing and doing their own thing. It takes patience, good directions, and a loud voice to lead successful group sessions for kids. Here are some ways to make the principles of water yoga fun and age-appropriate. These are short ideas that you can add into other aquatics programming as water yoga taste tests, or use as a base to build an entire water yoga class for kids.

Philosophy: Turn learning the names of the Yamas and Niyamas into alphabet soup. Everyone makes up a pose in the shape of the letter they're assigned. Once you spell the word, make sure to explain what it means.

Poses: Make poses partner poses by giving each pair of kids a noodle. They each hold the noodle in one hand and have to stay connected as they move through a series of postures. It's even more silly to ask them to stick their big toes in one end of the noodle and ask them to stay connected in that way. Unlike adults, kids love practicing inversions. Use handstands, headstands, Scorpion pose, Down Dog pose, and legs up the wall.

Breathwork: Who can stay underwater and make the biggest bubbles blowing out air? Or who can hold their breath the longest? Kids love taking turns being the judge.

Chanting: Have the kids chant underwater. In addition to chanting a regular Om, can they chant with a fish face or sounding like a whale? Have the kids create a customized class mantra to use each time you meet.

Meditation: Kids really get a kick out of a floating candle. Knowing it will blow out if submerged, they'll settle down to do a brief Trataka, or candle-gazing, meditation. During floating meditation, have the kids hold on to a buddy with one hand to become one long chain. I call it a sea otter float because they're all trying to take care of each other, so none of the baby sea otters get swept out to sea.

Turn yoga into a game! These are some kids water yoga games I've used:

Pool noodle jousting: Give each kid two pool noodles. The kids ride one noodle, and the other is their lance. They "trot" around on their noodles (which is a seated swim) and try and knock each other off.

Arch fish: Form two lines with the kids facing each other. Each person holds up one end of a noodle, forming a lined archway. Each yogi fish gets to swim through.

Royalty trust circle: The "king" and "queen" are in the center of a circle with their eyes closed. They fall, but the peasants on the outside catch them and set them back upright.

Lobster races: Kids put one noodle behind their back under their armpits. They have to swim backward like lobsters, and the fastest wins.

Floating yoga stations: Paint some boat fenders, or other floating objects, in different colors. Tether the fenders to something (buckets filled with rocks or kettle balls), so they float on the surface but don't float away. The kids have to perform a certain posture at each station.

Follow the leader: One person is in charge and picks the poses. They move through the pool, and everyone else follows along.

Yogi freeze tag: One kid is the shark. The shark swims around. If the shark tags you, you become stuck to the pool floor like seaweed (Tree pose). You can only "unfreeze" if another non-shark touches you.

Thread the needle: Form any of the standing postures with everyone facing the center of the circle. The kids take turns swimming through the circle of legs.

Hopscotch: Use recycled inner tubes. Fill the tubes with water, so they sink. Set up the hopscotch course. Use kids' dive toys for the marker. Have them "throw" the marker with their feet instead of their hands. The rest of the game is the same.

Householder/Grihastha stage
Water yoga for pregnancy
Pregnancy is a normal part of the human experience. Unless a woman has received special instructions from her doctor, she can participate in water yoga with the usual considerations for prenatal students. Apply the same modification considerations in water yoga as for prenatal land yoga:

- No breath retentions or aggressive breathing practices that could affect the oxygen supply to the baby.
- No low twists like Revolved Triangle or seated twists. There isn't room in the woman's torso, and they can apply too much pressure to the abdomen.

- No deep back arcs such as Camel because they can overstretch the abdominal muscles.
- No aggressive abdominal strengtheners like seated Leg Lifts as they can strain or damage the abdominal muscles.

Lying prone/supine in the water doesn't apply pressure to the body like a land-based environment. It's an okay position for poses like Plank or floating meditations if it doesn't bother your students. Unlike land-based yoga, there's no risk of overheating in a regular recreational pool. Pregnant women should not do water yoga in a hot tub.

Areas for emphasis that can help pregnant women make this life transition include postures that support hip and pelvic floor health like Goddess pose and Warrior II. Also, any of the stress management tools of water yoga, such as yoga philosophy, breathwork, and meditation, are very helpful to learn during pregnancy and can be carried into a woman's life with her baby.

Water yoga post-partum

Before resuming water yoga, a woman should be cleared by her healthcare professional for exercise. If, as a result of her pregnancy, she experiences incontinence, she'll need to work with her healthcare team to resolve that before resuming aquatic activities. Continue to avoid abdominal work if a woman has diastasis recti post-partum.

Water yoga for arthritis

There is very solid research on the benefits of both aquatic exercise and yoga for people living with arthritis. One of the most important things we can do for our students who live with arthritis is to help them build strength. Yes, that includes our traditional assumptions of muscular strength, since strong muscles support weak joints, but it also includes other aspects of strength such as cardiovascular endurance, resilience to stress or pain, and self-knowledge. Thinking of strength in its broadest terms, including the mind-body techniques and not just the poses, is important for this population.

Our limbs are basically a system of levers. Physics tells us a lever is a rigid bar (our bones), that moves at a fulcrum (our joints). There are two different forces that act on a lever (bone): resistance and effort. Resistance is what you're moving against, such as the water, and effort is the muscular contraction required to move. The fulcrum (joint) is the pivot point the motion happens at.

There are three kinds of levers. Most of the movements of our body are third class levers. That means when you bend your elbow to bring your palm to your shoulder in a biceps curl, there's resistance from the water against your hand, while your elbow is bending and your biceps muscle is creating the effort.

Raising the leg while it's straight or with a bent knee are both third class lever movements at the hip. However, the straight leg raise is asking the hip joint and your muscles to work harder. The resistance created by your foot is further from the hip joint (fulcrum). Plus, the increased surface area of the straight leg against the water increases the resistance from the water and makes the movement harder. Long lever movements require more effort, and create more joint load, than short lever movements. Using a buoyant prop, especially far away from the fulcrum joint, such as a pool noodle under the ankle in a straight leg lift, amplifies this effect.

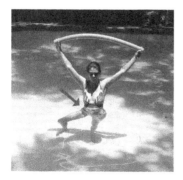 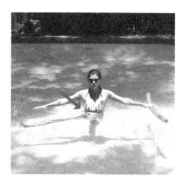

Short lever vs. long lever movements

Keep this principle in mind to tailor the workload for your students with arthritis. The goal of muscular strength building with arthritis is to load the muscles without joint strain so always use the appropriate size lever.

People who live with the autoimmune forms of arthritis face a significantly greater risk of coronary artery disease and heart failure. Increasing cardiovascular fitness is even more critical for this population than the average person. Use the more active, aerobic water yoga practices to improve heart health for these students.

Water yoga for multiple sclerosis (MS)

People with MS can participate in classes at the appropriate skill level for them like any other individual. The chief benefits from water yoga for people with MS are the improvements in balance, strengthening neural networks, and the opportunity to exercise without overheating.

Retiree/Vanaprastha stage
Water yoga for osteoporosis

Many women over 50 have osteopenia or osteoporosis. Aquatic exercise does not load joints as vigorously as land exercise due to buoyancy, but gains can still be made. The nature of the postures in water yoga makes the discipline very safe for people living with reduced bone density. The majority are standing and don't involve extreme forward flexion, twisting, or weight-bearing in the neck, which are areas of concern in land yoga with osteoporosis.

Water yoga for joint replacements

Always make sure people are cleared by their healthcare provider for physical/aquatic exercise before working with them after a joint replacement. Most of the people you will see will be months or years post-op and be very stable.

Joint replacements and water yoga

PROCEDURAL CONSIDERATIONS	WATER YOGA CONSIDERATIONS
ANTERIOR TOTAL HIP REPLACEMENT	
• Considered minimally invasive and currently more common • The piriformis, tensor fasciae latae, and sartorius muscles are cut	• No extensor stretches like Locust • No external rotation of the thighs/hips such as the leading leg in Warrior II • Do poses to one side only while healing
POSTERIOR TOTAL HIP REPLACEMENT	
• The gluteus muscles are split or cut • The piriformis and superior gemelli muscles are detached • The sciatic nerve can be damaged (rare)	• No adduction movements, especially crossing the legs • Limited hip flexion while healing (never greater than 90 degrees when healing so no Standing Pigeon)
KNEE REPLACEMENT	
• Multiple types of procedure available	• While healing avoid lateral stress such as eggbeater swirling actions • The knee's range of motion will be affected
ANKLE FUSION	
• Fusion of two or more ankle joints	• Will reduce ankle flexion like in Chair pose
ANKLE REPLACEMENT	
• Artificial joint replacement is the most common	• Often leads to permanent external rotation of the ankle so cue appropriately

Renunciate/Sannyas stage

Using the yoga sutras as guidance, the Renunciate stage is where we integrate all the information and practices from the first three chapters of the sutras and focus on detachment from the worldly environment.

In B.K.S. Iyengar's translations of the yoga sutras, he cites Lord Krishna's words to Arjuna from the Bhagavad Gita to describe this stage of life. The characteristics of a perfect yogi are, "Just as waters flow into the ocean, yet the level of the ocean neither changes nor becomes ruffled, similarly he who is steadfast in intelligence, pleasures do not haunt him, he attains liberation."

Panchamaya Kosha model

Like the ocean has layers, yoga philosophy tells us we have layers within ourselves working from the outer to inner. The last aspect of yoga philosophy relevant to water yoga is the Panchamaya Kosha model. The layers, or sheaths, in the Panchamaya Kosha model and what they represent, are:

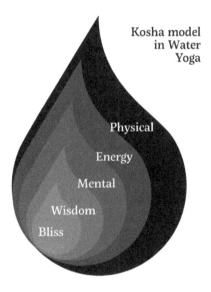

Annamaya: The physical sheath which is concerned with the part of our body we see and touch.

Pranamaya: The energy sheath which we impact with our breath.

Manomaya: The mental/emotional sheath where we process information, and figure out how to relate to the world.

Vijnanamaya: The wisdom sheath that holds our intuition.

Anandamaya: The bliss sheath where the most perfect, essential part of everything that makes us, us, resides.

Using an ocean analogy, we're most familiar with the splash zone, which we interact with at the seashore. The deep benthic zone at the bottom of the unexplored sea is harder to get to and less well known. Just like exploring the seven seas, most people find interacting with the outermost more physical Kosha layers easier than the innermost.

People like systems because they help us organize information. The Kosha model is a system that explains how to keep your body, mind, and spirit in optimal health. In science, the process your body uses to stay in a neutral, stable, functional place is called homeostasis. Just like being dehydrated sets off a chain of events within your biology to bring you back into homeostasis, living your life entirely in your physical sheath with no concern for your thoughts, feelings, or varying energy levels will set off a chain reaction that's guaranteed to get your attention in some way. A healthy body has all the sheaths functioning together.

On a practical level, a well-designed water yoga class reaches people on all levels of their being. Students engage with their physical body in an aquatic environment. They're learning anatomy, how to modify poses, and how to use props. Their energy body is stimulated by their breathwork practice. Or, if you implement any of the ideas from the Chakras into your class, that impacts the Pranayama sheath. Even the simplest Pratyahara practice, hydrostatic pressure, and meditation encourage awareness of the mental/emotional body. Whatever aspects of yoga philosophy you share touch people's wisdom body. Lastly, people can connect with their bliss body by dovetailing their spiritual practices with a water yoga practice, or chanting and vocalizations that integrate everything they've done in class.

How might the Kosha model vary throughout people's life stages? Kids are all about moving and are bundles of energy. While we might call a few kids "old souls," spiritual connection is not top in the mind for most kids. It's natural as people move through their life stages to more fully interact with all the layers of the Koshas. A person on the other end of the stages, in the Renunciate phase, might be focused on gearing their water yoga practice towards the spiritual and the bliss sheath.

The Panchamaya Kosha model is central to the field of yoga therapy. However, some people in the yoga therapy realm substitute or combine the Kosha model with the biopsychosocial model. The advantage to the biopsychosocial model is that it includes the importance of a social component to people's health.

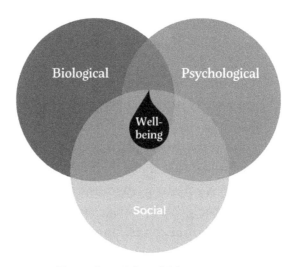

Biopsychosocial model in water yoga

The Kosha model doesn't include the beneficial impacts from strong social connections that people get from group aquatics classes. However, as soon as we put the Kosha model in the pool, we get the best of both systems.

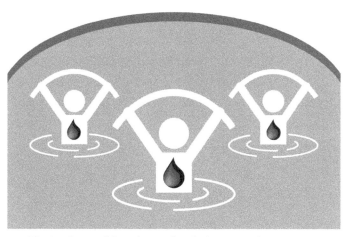

The Kosha model in the pool includes a social component

Most importantly, whatever age or stage your students are at, you're teaching the whole person. Be aware of where your students are in their life journeys. Know a few basic precautions for common health conditions. Integrate the Koshas to reinforce what your students need from water yoga. You're teaching group classes made up of unique individuals. Use these approaches to keep your teaching geared towards all aspects of your audience.

— Chapter 13 —

Inferred Benefits from Water Yoga

People come to wellness disciplines like water yoga because they want solutions to problems they're having, like nagging back pain, being overstressed, or feeling weak. In this case, people solve their problems by implementing water yoga. Some of their complaints are handled by the simple act of immersion. Everyone has physiological effects from immersion. The aquatic exercise component is another part of the puzzle with some unique benefits. Yoga, as a discipline, adds more benefits to the equation. People get closest to solving their problems with water yoga because it adds the effects of immersion to the benefits from aquatics and yoga, to offer a well-rounded solution to their needs.

Yoga as a system has lasted so long because it has helped so many people. Being able to communicate how it helps people as a professional is essential. Anecdotes and history are valuable, but when those things are combined with scientific research evidence, you can share the package of information with confidence.

Within this chapter, the term aquatics is used to mean head-out water exercise—things like aqua aerobics or aqua jogging. While I include swimming instructors and scuba divers as aquatic professionals interested in water yoga, those disciplines yield different research results. Since we don't get our face wet, or fully submerge in water yoga, that research is excluded from this discussion.

Top 11 most important physiological effects of immersion

The physiological effects of immersion lead to both certain benefits and cautions within water yoga. The results of immersion are based on solid science and apply to everyone when they reach the applicable depth. These 11 effects are the most important to know because they are the most relevant to your students during classes. The percentage of change to the body systems discussed varies depending on the temperature of the water you work in. However, the effects are still statistically significant across temperatures.

1. Being in the water increases heart efficiency

When you get in the water, more of your blood stays in your chest cavity, and your plasma volume increases. That means it's easier for your heart to move your blood around. Since beating got easier, your heart rate lowers. The increased efficiency carries over when you start to move. Consequently, your heart rate will stay lower when you're exercising in water rather than on land, and your muscles have an increased blood supply. Your lowered heart rate contributes to some of these other immersive effects related to the stress response below.

2. Immersion lowers blood pressure

The simple act of immersion lowers your blood pressure while you're in the water, and the effect continues for several hours after you're out of the pool. Aquatic exercise doubles this impact, as exercise, in general, reduces your normal blood pressure.

3. Getting in the water increases kidney efficiency

Immersing yourself in water increases the blood supply to your kidneys. That increase in blood supply makes your kidneys more efficient, and they increase their output. That increased output leads to greater excretions, which are higher in sodium and potassium. That's why aquatics classes are only 45 minutes on average. Most people really need to use the bathroom after 45 minutes in the water.

4. Immersion reduces edema (swelling)

The impact of the hydrostatic pressure and blood shifting into your thorax that occurs during immersion reduces swelling in your extremities. This helps people with reduced circulation, like diabetes, or people who struggle with blood pooling in their feet from injuries or pregnancy.

5. Getting in the water reduces fall risk

Falls are the leading cause of both fatal and non-fatal injuries for older adults. Pools are considered a low fall-risk environment because of the support of the water. You fall over in a slower and softer way in the water as oppposed to land, and you're less likely to get hurt if you do fall. I joke with my students if they fall in the water, the worst thing they're going to wound is their pride.

6. Being in the water modulates pain

Immersion alters people's interpretation of pain. When immersed, people's perception of pain is reduced. The water also increases people's pain tolerance. The leading theory is that both the water pressure and turbulence overload your pain sensory system. That's partly why people like hot tub jets.

7. Submersion decreases stress on joints.

Because of buoyancy, joints take less load in the pool. For people experiencing pain from musculoskeletal conditions such as arthritis, or an injury, that's a big help. Because you're more buoyant, your joints also have a little more space in them. Again, that reduces pain for people with arthritis and damaged joints.

That slight increase in space increases your range of motion in your joints by as much as 30 percent. For people with joint damage, this helps restore healthy movement. However, for experienced yogis, who may already be hypermobile, this can be dangerous. Performing water yoga poses allows you to put your body into shapes you may not be able to make on land. Make sure your students know that water yoga should challenge their muscles, but never cause joint pain.

8. Being in the water increases the relaxation response

Your relaxation response is another name for your autonomic nervous system (ANS). You might have heard it called the "rest and digest system." It controls many things, including heart rate, blood pressure, digestion, and breathing. As the name implies, your relaxation response is stimulated when you're relaxed. You can see there's a feedback loop with the water and your relaxation response. Because you like being in the water and it relaxes you, your ANS is stimulated. The bodily systems the ANS controls slow down. Because you're immersed, and immersion creates physiological changes, such as lowering your cortisol (the primary stress hormone) levels, that stimulates the relaxation response. Just like a relaxing bath, this effect may last for some time after getting out of the pool. However, for students who are afraid of the water, this effect may not be as robust.

9. Immersion increases heart rate variability

Heart rate variability (HRV) is the variation in time between your heartbeats. When you're healthy, your heart and nervous system can switch gears between being stressed and relaxed easily and quickly. Many different medical conditions reduce heart rate variability, and HRV has become a measurement of overall health. High heart rate variability is the goal for healthy individuals.

10. Being in the water strengthens respiratory muscles

One of the most powerful impacts of immersion, from a water yoga perspective, is that it strengthens your respiratory muscles. The hydrostatic pressure makes it harder to breathe in the water. Anyone with a breathing condition, such as COPD or asthma, benefits from stronger respiratory muscles. However, sudden immersion and the impacts of hydrostatic pressure can be too much and cause asthma or anxiety attacks. For anyone with this history, entering the water slowly is usually enough to prevent problems and enable them to still receive the benefits of immersion.

11. Being in the water decreases the thirst response

When you don't feel thirsty, you don't drink as much water. As a teacher, you want to encourage your students to stay hydrated. They don't realize that being in the water is actually dehydrating. Between the increased sodium and potassium output, and the decrease in water intake, people are also prone to muscle cramps in the pool. Encourage your students to hydrate in advance, and not get in the pool after just a morning cup of coffee. Use the bathroom, and drink water instead.

Benefits from aquatic exercise

The physiological effects of immersion strongly contribute to the benefits of aquatic exercise. While research has shown a broad swath of benefits from exercising in the water, here only those benefits that research has linked to aquatic exercise programs, and haven't been shown in yoga-based programs, are highlighted. These are related to the unique properties of moving while in the water.

Aquatic exercise improves exercise compliance

Your students might be coming to your class because they've been lectured by a healthcare provider about not getting enough exercise. Overall, physical activity is down across the board for us as humans. There are many reasons why that's the case, but research shows that people are more likely to stick with an aquatics exercise program than a land-based one. They see aquatic exercise as more fun and less painful, and perceive it as less effort than land exercise. Any exercise regime that your students are more likely to do is a win.

Aquatic exercise helps people stay cool while exercising

Water yoga is an exercise modality that doesn't involve overheating. It's vital for some people, such as pregnant ladies or people who live with multiple sclerosis, to not raise body temperature when exercising. Because aqua yoga is done in comfortably warm pools but isn't very aerobic, it keeps people's body temperature in a normal range.

Aquatic exercise reduces exercise-induced inflammation
Exercise-induced inflammation is the physical stress, strain, and potentially injury people experience from exercise. People experience less exercise-induced inflammation from aquatic exercise. That means that all people are not as sore after exercising in the water compared to land-based classes. It also means that anyone who lives with an inflammatory condition, such as fibromyalgia or systemic lupus erythematosus, is less likely to experience a systemic inflammatory response from their water exercise.

Aquatic exercise increases social engagement
People feel more socially engaged in an aquatics program. Because pool environments are louder and more public, they're not as quiet as a yoga studio. People feel more comfortable talking to others as they come and go from the pool, in the locker room, and potentially during their practice. It can be a more comfortable place to form social connections and make friends. Social engagement has a huge impact on health outcomes.

What benefits can we infer from water yoga?
There's a lot more public awareness about yoga these days. The average person on the street would describe yoga as increasing flexibility and reducing stress. Research solidly backs up public opinion in this case, and there are lots of resources out there for land yoga. Instead, we're focusing on the benefits of aquatics first, since the element of water is integral to the practice, then looking for the overlaps shown between the benefits of aquatics and yoga.

These are benefits that research has shown you get from both an aquatics program and a yoga practice. They speak to the practice's blended nature and the potential for even greater advantages to water yoga than either discipline alone.

However, as aqua yoga is an emerging discipline, we're not quite there yet. Immersion science does give us a solid place to start, but there is no existing water yoga research. Any potential benefits below are inferences from existing yoga and aquatics research. Aquatics research has expanded in the last 20 years along with yoga research, and we'll get there eventually. Keep that point in mind, and be clear when communicating with your students that these are only *potential* benefits.

Increase breath capacity
Some people believe that the entire point of yoga is breathing. Everyone at least agrees it's integral to the practice, and research has shown that breath practices performed in yoga increase breath capacity. Because immersion alone strengthens the respiratory muscles, it stands to reason that one of the biggest benefits of aqua yoga is an increase in breath capacity.

Reduce pain
Immersing a body reduces pain in multiple ways. Yoga teaches people how to manage the psychological components of pain by increasing pain management skills, such as reducing the incidence of pain catastrophizing. The two disciplines combined can provide a low-pain physical environment, with a highly functional pain-management attitude, for potentially combined benefits.

Slow the effects of aging
Leisure activities that help maintain physical fitness through the course of life reduce mortality. Any hobby with a physical component helps you age well. Aqua yoga might fulfill that benefit for many people.

Improve your overall health
Aquatic exercise has been shown to improve various health markers such as strength, balance, obesity, and quality of life. Yoga has shown similar benefits. In combining both benefits, aqua yoga may lead to general improvements in overall health.

Reduce chronic inflammation

Both being in the water and yoga have been shown to reduce various inflammatory markers in participants. This is potentially helpful for anyone who lives with diseases with a chronic inflammatory component, such as auto-immune conditions.

Build strength

Working in the water is challenging because of the water's resistance. You're using your muscles during a physical yoga practice. Doing aqua yoga probably builds strength too.

Create a balanced muscular effort

Because of the water's viscosity, you exert muscular effort in every direction when moving through the water. On land, you only build strength when moving against gravity. For example, biceps curls on land (without a weight) will build more biceps muscles than triceps muscles. In the water, you'll build both muscles equally if you exert equal pressure against the water in both directions.

Yoga creates balanced muscular effort better than other land exercise disciplines because of the yoga philosophy. Balance is a guiding principle of yoga. That's why you're encouraged to perform movements in both directions. When the disciplines are combined in aqua yoga, the balanced muscular effort may carry through.

Make people smarter

The increased efficiency of the heart when a person is in the water means the brain receives more oxygen. In aquatics, it's been shown to increase memory. With yoga, the discipline improves reaction times and accuracy. Combining both benefits, aqua yoga might stimulate even more of the brain.

To improve a person's mood

Both aquatics and yoga have been shown to improve mood states. Who doesn't want to be in a good mood? Aqua yoga might be a powerful modality for making people happier.

To reduce stress

Aquatic exercise can increase self-efficacy and decrease anxiety. Yoga teaches these and other stress management tools through yoga philosophy and meditation. Combining both disciplines, aqua yoga may yield even greater reductions in stress.

To increase relaxation

Just the act of immersion has a massive impact on your relaxation response. Yoga's impact on the autonomic nervous system is one of the leading exercise research areas right now because of the positive effects already found. This may be another area where aqua yoga yields significant improvements.

To improve confidence

The water is a great equalizer. Those with limitations can succeed in the same program as those who are more able-bodied on land. That increase in capabilities boosts people's confidence. It also hides things people don't like to show. You have to get in your suit, but other people can't see you once you're in the water. The anonymity makes people more comfortable. They can focus on what they're capable of, instead of what they look like when doing it. Aqua yoga also builds confidence by focusing on capabilities over limitations.

To improve balance

Both aquatics and yoga have been shown to improve the balance of participants. The act of standing on one leg, for example, builds both proprioceptive skills and muscular strength. Aqua yoga may be another way to increase balance through resisting buoyancy while performing aqua yoga poses.

To improve posture

Both aquatics and yoga strengthen the postural muscles in the back. Yoga adds stretching to lengthen the postural muscles that are constricted. The combined effect of stretching where you're tight and strengthening your weak areas leads to better postural alignment.

To improve postural control

Your posture is your ability to maintain the natural curves of your spine. Your balance is the ability to stay on your feet without falling over. Postural control is your body's ability to manage sensory input and keep your torso over your feet, so you don't fall. The three work together. Both aquatics and yoga improve your postural control by teaching you where your body is in space. Aqua yoga may do this in an even more powerful way.

To increase neuroplasticity

Neuroplasticity is about your brain's ability to create and organize neural connections. It's what allows you to learn new skills or to recover after an injury. Both yoga and aquatics have been shown to increase neuroplasticity biomarkers in participants. Combining the increase in neuroplasticity biomarkers with learning a new skill like aqua yoga may lead to increased neuroplasticity overall.

To reduce both the incidence of falls and their severity

Just being in the water reduces the possibility of falls that lead to injury. Reducing both the incidence and severity of falls makes falling less risky overall. Participating in aquatics or yoga leads to better balance through greater strength and body awareness, which reduces the incidence of falls when on land.

While these water yoga benefits are inferences at this time, it is hoped that in the future there will be solid research on water yoga that will allow us to address the subject in a more concrete way. In the meantime, these are the things that matter to your students. These potential benefits are what makes their lives better and why they come to class. Share this information with your students, but be honest about the strength of the claims.

Chapter 14

Water Yoga Safety and Comfort

While water yoga overall is a very safe way to practice yoga, there are always special safety considerations when working around water. These are some tips and tricks to keep you as a teacher, and your students, safe and comfortable during water yoga.

Best places to practice and teach water yoga

The best place to practice water yoga is in a swimming pool because it's the most reliable. Using a hot tub, lake, and the ocean also work, but each has its safety considerations.

Public or private swimming pools: These are usually the easiest, most consistent option. Use the shallow end where the bottom is flat, and the water is mid-chest height. You typically have no control over the temperature of the pool, so choose locations that meet your needs and adjust your classes appropriately. A pool temperature of 82 to 85 degrees Fahrenheit is ideal for aqua yoga. When under 80 degrees, such as the temperature of pools for competitive swimming, you'll have to work hard as a teacher to keep people warm.

Therapy temperature pool: If you're using a very warm pool (over 85 degrees Fahrenheit), students can overheat. That's especially true for pregnant ladies or people with certain medical conditions like multiple sclerosis. If it's a warm outdoor pool, do yoga in the shady side, if possible. You can shift your practice times to mornings or evenings when it's cooler. If it's available, position yourself to take advantage of a breeze.

Hot tub: Students are even more prone to overheating in a hot tub. Make sure their doctor has cleared them to be in the hot tub, and keep the sessions shorter. People are able to stretch further than normal in such warm water. When using a hot tub, emphasize that students need to stop in a posture before reaching their full end range of motion, and listen to their bodies.

Lakes/rivers: It's possible to do water yoga in a lake as long as the bottom is good enough to work with. A lot of lakes have muddy or rocky bottoms which are too uncomfortable to stand on. As long as the footing is firm and stable, and the water is warm enough, your students will be fine.

Ocean: When working on a beach, try to choose one that doesn't have waves or a lot of swell, and be aware of the tides. The depth of the water on any given day might vary considerably. Use a tide chart to help you plan, if relevant. If the beach has a slope, you'll need to adjust all the positions to accommodate that. It's easier for people to work with their heels facing downhill but that might position students so their back is to the incoming waves. Never turn your back on the ocean. If doing a pose in one direction requires you to place your back foot (the downhill foot) so that you're facing away from the water, spin yourself around. Always face the water with the back foot downhill. You can use the ebb and flow of the water as part of the timing of your arm movements and to emphasize breathwork practice. Most importantly, never get in the ocean alone.

Before teaching at a location for the first time, always get in the pool or other body of water yourself and check out the bottom. Then, you can inform your students of slick or unlevel spots, or visibility concerns, and so on.

The ingress/egress areas of pools can get crowded with gear. Encourage students to stow their swim bags/shoes away from the pool edge. Students who use mobility aids need them as close as possible to the entrance/exit of the pool to assist them. Still, you may need to move walkers or canes back and forth for easy access for your students while keeping the area safe for others.

Water safety

Should you teach from the pool deck or in the water with your students? The answer is: it depends. According to the Aquatic Exercise Association, the best practice is for instructors to teach from the pool deck. That allows you to see all your students well, be able to get to students fast should they have a safety issue, and allows students to see you well. However, students at the back can't hear you, and it's hard to demonstrate some of the poses accurately. Also, you can't physically help an individual student. In summary, always teach from the pool deck if there's no lifeguard on duty, or you need to practice social distancing.

Teaching while in the pool is good when you need to offer a lot of individualized attention, especially in a private session. Other good reasons to teach in the water include teaching a sequence with a lot of suspended poses, or when you need to protect your own body as a teacher.

Know all the rules of the pool you're teaching in. That might be as simple as whatever the owner tells you, or it might be a book of procedures for a municipal pool. Know the emergency action plan for the pool you work at and always follow the instructions of the lifeguards.

Whatever body of water you're in, practice lightning safety. You can get a free lightning app for your phone to help you stay safe or remember the adage "When thunder roars, get indoors." If you're practicing in a public pool, always follow all the lightning protocols.

Stay hydrated! Being in the water is more dehydrating than people think. Your kidneys are cycling more efficiently because of hydrostatic pressure. You're using fluids faster internally even though you're all wet. Encourage students to keep a water bottle on the pool deck to use during class or to keep one in their swim bag for after class. Using a metal water bottle is also safer than glass, and better for you and the planet than plastic.

Communicate to your students the basic contraindications for engaging in aquatic activity—no open wounds or skin infections, no incontinence, no diarrhea, and no urinary tract infections.

Have your students rinse off before they get in the pool. You should as well if you're teaching in the water. It removes sweat and personal care products, which keep the water quality high for everyone's sake.

If there are lots of bugs around, it's not good for the water quality to wear bug spray. It would be better to shift the time of day you practice or borrow a screened-in pool, if possible.

Personal care for your students

I find students get more benefits from water yoga without shoes, but that's not a choice for everyone. Students should absolutely wear shoes if they've been told to by a doctor, have diabetes and/or neuropathy, or are worried about slipping.

Always encourage students to think about sun protection. Share best practices from dermatologists such as wearing sunscreen and UV sun clothes. In addition, remember sunglasses and hats.

Staying warm in the pool is sometimes a more significant issue than sun protection. UV clothes also work as insulators to help people stay warm. There are also insulated swimwear options. Head coverings such as hats and swim caps also help people stay warm. Some women also want to wear hair coverings to keep their hair dry, or covered for modesty. Swim clothes should always be made of the appropriate fabric. Cotton is not good for water quality, and that's why it's banned in pools.

Some women find the water and chlorine overly drying to their mucus membranes, which can result in vaginitis and other infections. A personal lubricant that does not contain glycerin can help. Some women find wearing a tampon in the pool helps prevent "drying out" as well.

After being in the pool, students need to take care of their hair and skin. Everyone should always rinse to remove the chlorine. There are commercial rinses that work for both hair and skin, so you don't have to carry multiple bottles. Look for a brand that contains Vitamin C as that naturally neutralizes chlorine. After the chlorine is off, remember to moisturize.

Muscle cramps during water yoga, especially in the feet and lower legs, are common when people start. Those small muscles get fatigued and overloaded from all the new ways they're being used. The problem usually goes away after six weeks because students gain strength in their feet and calves. Encourage good hydration and a visit to their healthcare provider if the problem persists.

The same rules regarding exertion in land yoga apply to a water yoga practice. When practicing water yoga postures, students should always practice within their personal limits. You can tell your students, "It's okay to have sensations and feel a stretch when practicing. If you feel your practice the next day, that's okay too. If you're sore for more than 24 hours after practicing, you pushed too hard, and you need to back off next time."

Personal care and safety for you

- Always use sun protection. Outdoor pools might have sun umbrellas you can teach under to protect your skin and stay cool.
- To protect your skin, after practicing use a chlorine neutralizer rinse. There are do-it-yourself recipes online if you'd rather make your own than buy one.

- Keep yourself hydrated, especially when teaching from the pool deck. Build in a water break with your cues by saying things like "repeat that movement three more times on each side."
- Protect your voice. Stay hydrated. Breathe deeply to project well. Don't shout over competing activities in the pool. Ask if others can be quieter or if accessories like mushrooms and splash baskets can be turned off while you teach. Use a microphone, if available. Use your hands in place of words. You can use your fingers to count down repetitions instead of verbally repeating directions, for example.
- Wear shoes on the pool deck. They protect your feet, and stop you from slipping. Some pools have mats for instructors. Teaching on one will save wear and tear on your body while demonstrating.

Gear safety

- Check any gear you're going to be using before you start. Noodles wear out fast when left out in the sun, and the handles of dumbbells can become uncomfortable.
- Remember that buoyant props are not flotation or lifesaving aids.
- Know the pool's policy about bringing in outside gear. For example, most pools ban monofins. Do they have any rules that will impact you?
- Always have a spare set of equipment for what you're teaching. Things can break in the middle of class, or people show up late.

Business safety

Make sure you have met the regulatory, legal, and insurance rules for your area, such as making sure your students are signing liability waivers. A valuable tip is to include a photo release on your liability forms so that you can share pictures of your classes in your marketing materials. Consult with a local professional, or your business development office, if you need help with the requirements where you teach.

Public pools have lifeguards, but in a private pool, you are not the guard unless you have that qualification also. Ensure that all students know they're using the pool at their own risk when there is no guard. Keep your previously charged cell phone nearby when teaching in case of emergencies.

These tips will help you keep yourself and your students safe and healthy for the long term. Safety is sometimes regarded as boring but that's really not true. A safe practice is a fun practice. Harmful accidents are never fun and are almost always preventable. How can you borrow some principles from the pro bike helmet "Safety is Sexy" campaign? Instead of "No, you can't," make your teaching, "Yes, you can, like this…"

— Chapter 15 —

Moving Forward with Water Yoga

This is it, your last kick turn, in your last lap of reading about water yoga. You've been swimming through the idea of the eight waves of water yoga and now you're on the last one, Samadhi. You started with yoga philosophy and the Yamas, or restraints, moving into the second wave with the Niyamas, or observances. Those mental practices prepared your attitude for Samadhi. You spent more than one lap dealing with the third wave, Asanas. Pranayama, the fourth wave, focused on breathwork. The third and fourth waves prepared your body for Samadhi. The fifth wave, Pratyahara, or withdrawing your senses, transitioned you to the sixth and seventh waves, Dharana and Dhyana. Those were concentration and meditation respectively, which taught you how to deal with your energy and focus.

This last and eighth wave of water yoga is Samadhi. Samadhi is about integrating all aspects of a water yoga practice to help you achieve a higher plane of consciousness above the mundane activities in the pool. There's no worrying about the past, the future, or anything outside your control. You are totally absorbed in your activities. It makes sense that this is the goal of a water yoga practice because who doesn't want a life filled with joy and bliss, free of stress?

You reach Samadhi by absorbing yourself in Dharana and Dhyana. In Dharana, you sharpened your focus towards one thing. In meditation, every time your mind wandered, you brought it back to your one thing. In Samadhi, your distractions have ceased. The barriers between you and the point of your concentration have softened and dissolved. It's that place where there is no barrier between where your body ends, and the water begins. You're connected not just to yourself, but to the fluid energy around you.

While fusing the best version of yourself with the power of the universe through perfection in your water yoga practice sounds lovely, there's no guarantee you'll get there. You practice being attached to the process and not the results. The book has taught you the steps to create a water yoga practice and program, but you don't know where you'll end up on your journey. The book has only shown you the path you need to take. It's taught you how to organize the pathway for yourself and your students, so you're both more likely to hit Samadhi as your destination.

Water yoga is essentially a solitary experience. It's about integrating all aspects of yoga into your body. You're trying to effectively integrate all the sensory, energetic, and intellectual aspects of the practice for yourself. To be an effective teacher, you need to move past personal integration and develop synergy with your students.

From the dictionary, synergy is the combined power of a group of things that when working together will form a greater total power than they could have achieved by working separately. As humans, we crave community and connection, which is why public classes are so popular. The synergy created by sharing water yoga with others is more powerful than just personally integrating it.

By sharing, you're not approaching Samadhi by yourself. You're bringing others with you. It's like the idea that the rising tide raises all boats. You're taking your yoga out into the world and empowering others too. It goes beyond empowering yourself and expands your reach into the broader definitions of power. I'm a fan of the work of Brené Brown and I like the description of power she uses. Her definition, originally described by social worker Mary Parker Follett, lays out four components of power: power within, power to, power with, and power over.

Power over is about coercion and control. You've learned that it has no place in yoga, so we're discarding that and not exploring it any further.

Power within is the agency to be your best self and stand in your strength. You know your own worth and are comfortable in your own skin. Integrating all the tools of water yoga has given you power within yourself. Power within is the perfect description of the whole point of water yoga and reaching Samadhi within your personal practice.

Power to is sharing your power to bring others up with you. It's focused on sharing your knowledge and learning. It calls on you to be like the gurus who have shared yoga through the ages. Yoga has actually always taken place in a group setting. Each person was an individual practitioner, but they learned from a guru in a Shala, a community, or home, for yoga.

Power to is built on the synergy you create with your students. It helps others see the power you've built within and shows them how to create the same power within themselves. You do not diminish your power by sharing, you make the entire community more powerful. Samadhi by yourself is lonely. How can you bring others up with you on your journey?

Integration plus synergy equals growth. Growth for everyone is the heart of power with. Power with is acknowledging the inherent agency in each of us. Together you are collaborating in solidarity to effect change in yourselves and your community. It is the most inherently yogic method of sharing the principles of yoga. It makes water yoga not just a sensory experience for yourself, or a benefit for people who already use the pool, but a possibility for everyone.

Power with inspired women early in the 20th century to push for a shift in societal standards around women and sport. Modest bathing wear was a safety hazard. It literally kept women out of the water. By shifting the conversation from what couldn't be seen to what could be accomplished, women have shown they're actually superior at ultra long-distance swims.

Power with provided a forum for African Americans to demand

access to public swimming pools in the 1960s. White and black swimmers staged "swim-ins" together. The most impactful occurred in St. Augustine, Florida, and contributed to the signing of the 1964 Civil Rights Act.

These struggles continue to be relevant today in the discussion around making diverse head coverings acceptable in all levels of aquatic activities. Olympics athletes have faced discrimination for wearing swim caps that cover dreadlocks. Women wanting to cover their hair and/or bodies for religious reasons have faced discrimination at local pools.

As water yoga teachers, we can use power with to be leaders in our communities. We can create a culture of power with that makes everyone welcome in the pool. We can provide instruction that is inclusive of people of all abilities. We can empower others to share water yoga with their friends and family.

If that seems pie in the sky, think about ways to make it real. Provide scholarships to your classes, apply for grants to underwrite whole programs, mentor other professionals who represent different communities than you. When you apply power with to a growth mindset, the limiting factor is not creativity. Water yoga has taught you Tapas, so you have the will. You just need to create the way.

That growth will bring more people to water yoga. More people will get the benefits of the practice. That, in turn, will create more demand for classes, and both your business and the field will grow. Your water yoga offerings are the proverbial pebble that ripples out. But you're not tossing a pebble into a puddle—the ripples from what you do will spread through your pool and community because others are tossing in their pebbles too.

Water always follows the path of least resistance, yet its flowing energy can change a landscape. I've broken down the barriers for you and shown you the water yoga path to Samadhi. It's up to you to travel it and bring others with you, so you can change your landscape together.

Notes

Introduction
O'Grady, P. (n.d.). Thales of Miletus. *Internet Encyclopedia of Philosophy*. https://iep.utm.edu/thales.

Chapter 1
Basavaraddi, I. (2015, April 23). *Yoga, its origin history and development*. Ministry of External Affairs, Government of India. www.mea.gov.in/in-focus-article.htm?25096%2FYoga%2BIts%2BOrigin%2BHistory%2Band%2BDevelopment.

Chapter 2
Iyengar, B.K.S. (1993). *Light on Yoga, Sutras of Patanjali*. London: Thorsons.
Verne, J. (2020). *20,000 Leagues under the Sea*. Duke Classics.

Chapter 3
Aquatic Exercise Association (2018). *Aquatic Fitness Professional Manual*. Champaign, IL: Human Kinetics.

Chapter 5
Becker, B.E. & Cole, A.J. (1997). *Comprehensive Aquatic Therapy*. Philadelphia, PA: Butterworth-Heinemann.
Ma, X., *et al.* (2017). The effect of diaphragmatic breathing on attention, negative affect and stress in healthy adults. *Frontiers in Psychology*, 8, 874.
Porges, S.W. (2017). *The Pocket Guide to the Polyvagal Theory: The Transformative Power of Feeling Safe*. New York, NY: W.W. Norton & Company.
Saoji, A.A., Raghavendra, B.R., & Manjunath, N.K. (2019). Effects of yogic breath regulation: A narrative review of scientific evidence. *Journal of Ayurveda and Integrative Medicine*, 10(1), 50–58.

Chapter 6
Seale, A. (2016, October 24). *The Liminal Space*. Center for Transformational Presence. https://transformationalpresence.org/alan-seale-blog/liminal-space-embracing-mystery-power-transition-will-2.

Chapter 7

Mooventhan, A. & Khode, V. (2014). Effect of Bhramari pranayama and OM chanting on pulmonary function in healthy individuals: A prospective randomized control trial. *International Journal of Yoga*, 7(2), 104–110.

Quote Investigator (2020, July 21). "Whether you believe you can do a thing or not, you are right." https://quoteinvestigator.com/2015/02/03/you-can.

Swanson, A. (2019). *Science of Yoga: Understand the Anatomy and Physiology to Perfect Your Practice*. New York, NY: DK.

Zhu, J., Wekerle, C., Lanius, R., & Frewen, P. (2019). Trauma- and stressor-related history and symptoms predict distress experienced during a brief mindfulness meditation sitting: Moving toward trauma-informed care in mindfulness-based therapy. *Mindfulness*, 10(10), 1985–1996.

Chapter 8

Abbott A. (2017). Evaluating in introduction of Ai Chi to a pain management programme. *British Journal of Pain*, 11(1), 69–70.

Chaiopanont S. (2008). Hypoglycemic effect of sitting breathing meditation exercise on type 2 diabetes at Wat Khae Nok Primary Health Center in Nonthaburi Province. *Journal of the Medical Association of Thailand*, 91(1), 93–98.

Chan, R.R., Giardino, N., & Larson, J.L. (2015). A pilot study: mindfulness meditation intervention in COPD. *International Journal of Chronic Obstructive Pulmonary Disease*, 10, 445–454.

Feinstein, J.S., *et al.* (2018). Examining the short-term anxiolytic and antidepressant effect of Floatation-REST. *PloS One*, 13(2), e0190292.

Gainey, A., Himathongkam, T., Tanaka, H., & Suksom, D. (2016). Effects of Buddhist walking meditation on glycemic control and vascular function in patients with type 2 diabetes. *Complementary Therapies in Medicine*, 26, 92–97.

Goyal, M., *et al.* (2014). Meditation programs for psychological stress and well-being: a systematic review and meta-analysis. *JAMA Internal Medicine*, 174(3), 357–368.

Kjellgren, A. & Westman, J. (2014). Beneficial effects of treatment with sensory isolation in flotation-tank as a preventive health-care intervention: A randomized controlled pilot trial. *BMC Complementary Medicine and Therapies*, 14, 417.

Kurt, E.E., *et al.* (2018). Effects of Ai Chi on balance, quality of life, functional mobility, and motor impairment in patients with Parkinson's disease. *Disability and Rehabilitation*, 40(7), 791–797.

Plunket, B., Mooneyham, D.J., Hendry, R., & Walker, C. (n.d.). *Ai Chi*. RuthSova.com. http://ruthsova.com/ai-chi.

Robert-McComb, J.J., *et al.* (2015). The effects of mindfulness-based movement on parameters of stress. *International Journal of Yoga Therapy*, 25(1), 79–88.

Wu, L.L., Lin, Z.K., Weng, H.D., Qi, Q.F., Lu, J., & Liu, K.X. (2018). Effectiveness of meditative movement on COPD: A systematic review and meta-analysis. *International Journal of Chronic Obstructive Pulmonary Disease*, 13, 1239–1250.

Chapter 9

Rezai, V., Mahdavi-Nejad, R., & Zolaktaf, V. (2020). Comparing the effects of different types of aquatic walking on endurance and electrical activities of spine extensor muscles in men with nonspecific chronic back pain. *International Journal of Preventive Medicine*, 11, 168.

Whitworth, G. (2019, February 11). What is a normal respiratory rate? *Medical News Today*. www.medicalnewstoday.com/articles/324409.

Chapter 10

Pursuit of Happiness. (2021, February 13). *Abraham Maslow*. www.pursuit-of-happiness. org/history-of-happiness/abraham-maslow.

Chapter 11

Aquatic Exercise Association (2018). *Aquatic Fitness Professional Manual*. Champaign, IL: Human Kinetics.

Coronal: https://commons.wikimedia.org/wiki/File:Coronal.png.

Heyman, J. (2019). *Accessible Yoga*. Boulder, CO: Shambala.

Sagittal: https://commons.wikimedia.org/wiki/File:Sagittal.png.

Transverse: https://commons.wikimedia.org/wiki/File:Transverse.png.

Chapter 12

Bedekar, N., *et al.* (2012). Comparative study of conventional therapy and additional yoga-sanas for knee rehabilitation after total knee arthroplasty. *International Journal of Yoga*, 5(2), 118–122.

Bone Health and Osteoporosis Foundation (2021, July 17). *Exercise/safe movement*. www. bonehealthandosteoporosis.org/patients/treatment/exercisesafe-movement

Brearley, A.L., *et al.* (2015). Pregnant women maintain body temperatures within safe limits during moderate-intensity aqua-aerobic classes conducted in pools heated up to 33 degrees Celsius: An observational study. *Journal of Physiotherapy*, 61(4), 199–203.

Corvillo, I., *et al.* (2017). Efficacy of aquatic therapy for multiple sclerosis: a systematic review. *European Journal of Physical and Rehabilitation Medicine*, 53(6), 944–952.

Cramer, H., *et al.* (2014). Yoga for multiple sclerosis: A systematic review and meta-analysis. *PLoS One*, 9(11), e112414.

Crowson, C.S., *et al.* (2013). Rheumatoid arthritis and cardiovascular disease. *American Heart Journal*, 166(4), 622–628.

Desikachar, T.K.V. (1999). *The Heart of Yoga: Developing a Personal Practice*. Rochester, VT: Inner Traditions.

Eversden, L., *et al.* (2007). A pragmatic randomised controlled trial of hydrotherapy and land exercises on overall well being and quality of life in rheumatoid arthritis. *BMC Musculoskeletal Disorders*, 8, 23.

Fisken, A., *et al.* (2014). Perception and responses to different forms of aqua-based exercise among older adults with osteoarthritis. *International Journal of Aquatic Research and Education*, 8(1), 32–52.

Hertz, D.P. (2003). *Aquatic Exercise Programming for People with Multiple Sclerosis*. National MS Society.

Holden, S.C., *et al.* (2019). Prenatal yoga for back pain, balance, and maternal wellness: A randomized, controlled pilot study. *Global Advances in Health and Medicine*, Aug 26: 8.

Iyengar, B.K.S. (1993) *Light on Yoga, Sutras of Patanjali*. London: Thorsons (page 145).

Łyp, M., *et al.* (2016). A water rehabilitation program in patients with hip osteoarthritis before and after total hip replacement. *International Medical Journal of Experimental and Clinical Research*, 22, 2635–2642.

Mears, S.C., *et al.* (2019). Ankle motion in common yoga poses. *Foot*, 39, 55–59.

Moonaz, S.H. (2015). Yoga in sedentary adults with arthritis: Effects of a randomized controlled pragmatic trial. *Journal of Rheumatology*, 42(7),1194–1202.

Rodríguez-Blanque, R., *et al.* (2019). Randomized clinical trial of an aquatic physical exercise program during pregnancy. *Journal of Obstetric, Gynecologic & Neonatal Nursing*, 48(3), 321–331.

Simas V., *et al.* (2017). Effects of water-based exercise on bone health of middle-aged and older adults: A systematic review and meta-analysis. *Open Access Journal of Sports Medicine*, 8, 39–60.

Weigenfeld-Lahav, I., *et al.* (2007). Physical and psychological effects of aquatic therapy in participants after hip-joint replacement: A pilot study. *International Journal of Aquatic Research and Education*, 1, 2.

Chapter 13

Aquatic Exercise Association (2018). *Aquatic Fitness Professional Manual*. Champaign, IL: Human Kinetics.

Arnold, C.M. & Faulkner, R.A. (2010). The effect of aquatic exercise and education on lowering fall risk in older adults with hip osteoarthritis. *Journal of Aging and Physical Activity*, 18(3), 245–260.

Becker, B.E. & Cole, A.J. (1997). *Comprehensive Aquatic Therapy*. Philadelphia, PA: Butterworth-Heinemann.

Binkley, H.M. & Rudd, L.E. (2018). Head-out aquatic exercise for generally healthy postmenopausal women: A systematic review. *Journal of Physical Activity & Health*, 1–22.

Büssing, A., Ostermann, T., Lüdtke, R., & Michalsen, A. (2012). Effects of yoga interventions on pain and pain-associated disability: A meta-analysis. *The Journal of Pain*, 13(1), 1–9.

Crowe, B.M. & Van Puymbroeck, M. (2019). Enhancing problem- and emotion-focused coping in menopausal women through yoga. *International Journal of Yoga Therapy*, 29(1), 57–64.

de Oliveira, G., *et al.* (2016). Yoga training has positive effects on postural balance and its influence on activities of daily living in people with multiple sclerosis: A pilot study. *Explore*, 12(5), 325–332.

de Oliveira Ottone, V., *et al.* (2014). The effect of different water immersion temperatures on post-exercise parasympathetic reactivation. *PloS One*, 9(12), e113730.

Dong, R., *et al.* (2018). Is aquatic exercise more effective than land-based exercise for knee osteoarthritis? *Medicine*, 97(52), e13823.

Duda, D. (2011, August). *Water exercise: a cool (and easy) way to exercise*. MS Magazine. www.msfocusmagazine.org/Magazine/Magazine-Items/Posted/Water-Exercise-A-Cool-(and-Easy)-Way-to-Exercise.

Francis, A. & Beemer, R. (2019). How does yoga reduce stress? Embodied cognition and emotion highlight the influence of the musculoskeletal system. *Complementary Therapies in Medicine*, 43, 170–175.

Gautam, S., Tolahunase, M., Kumar, U., & Dada, R. (2019). Impact of yoga-based mind-body intervention on systemic inflammatory markers and co-morbid depression in active rheumatoid arthritis patients: A randomized controlled trial. *Restorative Neurology and Neuroscience*, 37(1), 41–59.

Gianesini, S., *et al.* (2017). A specifically designed aquatic exercise protocol to reduce chronic lower limb edema. *Phlebology*, 32(9), 594–600.

Glass, S.M., *et al.* (2018). Changes in posture following a single session of long-duration water immersion. *Journal of Applied Biomechanics*, 34(6), 435–441

Gothe, N., Pontifex, M.B., Hillman, C., & McAuley, E. (2013). The acute effects of yoga on executive function. *Journal of Physical Activity & Health*, 10(4), 488–495.

Gunay, S.M., Keser, I., & Bicer, Z.T. (2018). The effects of balance and postural stability exercises on spa based rehabilitation programme in patients with ankylosing spondylitis. *Journal of Back and Musculoskeletal Rehabilitation*, 31(2), 337–346.

Hakked, C.S., Balakrishnan, R., & Krishnamurthy, M.N. (2017). Yogic breathing practices improve lung functions of competitive young swimmers. *Journal of Ayurveda and Integrative Medicine*, 8(2), 99–104.

Hamrick, I., *et al.* (2017). Yoga's effect on falls in rural, older adults. *Complementary Therapies in Medicine*, 35, 57–63.

Kang, H.S., *et al.* (2007). Aquatic exercise in older Korean women with arthritis: Identifying barriers to and facilitators of long-term adherence. *Journal of Gerontological Nursing*, 33(7), 48–56.

Kargarfard, M., *et al.* (2018). Randomized controlled trial to examine the impact of aquatic exercise training on functional capacity, balance, and perceptions of fatigue in female patients with multiple sclerosis. *Archives of Physical Medicine and Rehabilitation*, 99(2), 234–241.

Kim, J.H., *et al.* (2018). Effects of aquatic and land-based exercises on amyloid beta, heat shock protein 27, and pulse wave velocity in elderly women. *Experimental Gerontology*, 108, 62–68.

Martínez-Carbonell Guillamón, E., *et al.* (2019). Does aquatic exercise improve commonly reported predisposing risk factors to falls within the elderly? A systematic review. *BMC Geriatrics*, 19(1), 52.

National Council on Aging (2021, July 14). *Get the Facts on Falls Prevention*. National Council on Aging. www.ncoa.org/article/get-the-facts-on-falls-prevention.

Pascoe, M.C., Thompson, D.R., & Ski, C.F. (2017). Yoga, mindfulness-based stress reduction and stress-related physiological measures: A meta-analysis. *Psychoneuroendocrinology*, 86, 152–168.

Pendergast, D.R., *et al.* (2015). Human physiology in an aquatic environment. *Comprehensive Physiology*, 5(4), 1705–1750.

Pérez-de la Cruz, S. (2019). Mental health in Parkinson's disease after receiving aquatic therapy: A clinical trial. *Acta Neurologica Belgica*, 119(2), 193–200.

Pires, D., Cruz, E.B., & Caeiro, C. (2015). Aquatic exercise and pain neurophysiology education versus aquatic exercise alone for patients with chronic low back pain: A randomized controlled trial. *Clinical Rehabilitation*, 29(6), 538–547.

Prado, E.T., *et al.* (2014). Hatha yoga on body balance. *International Journal of Yoga*, 7(2), 133–137.

Saint-Maurice, P.F., *et al.* (2019). Association of leisure-time physical activity across the adult life course with all-cause and cause-specific mortality. *JAMA Network Open*, 2(3), e190355.

Sherlock, L., Guyton, W., & Rye, J. (2013). The physiological effects of aquatic exercise on cognitive function in the aging population. *International Journal of Aquatic Research and Education*, 7(3), 266–278.

Silva, L., *et al.* (2019). Effects of aquatic exercise on mental health, functional autonomy and oxidative stress in depressed elderly individuals: A randomized clinical trial. *Clinics*, 74, e322.

Tolahunase, M.R., Sagar, R., Faiq, M., & Dada, R. (2018). Yoga- and meditation-based lifestyle intervention increases neuroplasticity and reduces severity of major depressive disorder: A randomized controlled trial. *Restorative Neurology and Neuroscience*, 36(3), 423–442.

Versey, N.G., Halson, S.L., & Dawson, B.T. (2013). Water immersion recovery for athletes: Effect on exercise performance and practical recommendations. *Sports Medicine (Auckland, N.Z.)*, 43(11), 1101–1130.

Chapter 15

"Brené Brown with Joe Biden on empathy, unity and courage." (2020, October 21). *Unlocking Us*. Spotify.

https://open.spotify.com/episode/2APKx5PPXL9Vls0tOjdLIe?go=1&utm_source=embed_v3&t=0&nd=1.

Diallo, R. (2021, April 21). *Opinion: France's latest vote to BAN hijabs shows how far it will go to exclude Muslim women*. The Washington Post. www.washingtonpost.com/opinions/2021/04/21/france-hijab-ban-vote-exclusion.

Navarrete, D. (2020, August 28). *Why women have beaten men in marathon swimming?* Swimming World News. www.swimmingworldmagazine.com/news/why-women-have-beaten-men-in-marathon-swimming.

NPR (2014, June 13). *Remembering a civil rights swim-in: "It was a milestone."* NPR. www.npr.org/2014/06/13/321380585/remembering-a-civil-rights-swim-in-it-was-a-milestone.

Owoseje, T. (2021, July 16). *FINA to review use of Afro swim cap at competition level after facing criticism*. CNN. www.cnn.com/2021/07/05/sport/fina-soul-cap-black-hair-olympics-spt-intl-scli-gbr/index.html.

Index

Page numbers in italics indicate illustrations.

About the Author

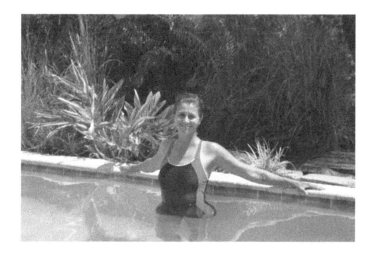

Christa Fairbrother, MA, ERYT 200/500, is an internationally recognized water yoga coach and trainer. She comes to teaching water yoga with a BFA from the University of Washington in metal design, an MA in museum education, and ten years of work experience as a farrier. Her creative approach to the practice comes from her artist's eye, her practical experience of improving movement on the job, and thirty years of practicing yoga. Her background in teaching in nontraditional environments makes her excel as a teacher's teacher. She lives with her husband and two sons in Florida. For more information, her website is www.christafairbrother.com.